A MAN DERAILED

Paul Holmes

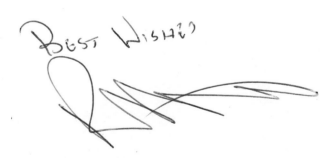

chipmunkapublishing

the mental health publisher

empowering people with depression

Paul Holmes

Published by

Chipmunkapublishing

PO Box 6872

Brentwood

Essex CM13 1ZT

United Kingdom

http://www.chipmunkapublishing.com

Copyright © Paul Holmes 2008

Edited by Angela Barsby

Chipmunkapublishing gratefully acknowledge the support of Arts Council England.

A MAN DERAILED

Thanks & Acknowledgements

I wish to thank Chipmunka Publishing for this amazing opportunity. Writing this book has been the best tool I could have had for fighting away the demons within. So to Jason Pegler and the rest of your team I thank you very much.

Thanks to my Mum & Dad for their amazing help and support in my wife & I's new life.

Thanks to Len & Stella for your support also.

I wish to thank Bruce (you're a crap counsellor mate but a bloody great friend. Please don't ever try and talk someone out of jumping from a roof). However, please don't ever change.

I wish to thank Good Companions in Southend for all the work they do.

I wish to thank Steve for dragging me around golf courses and watching me smash my clubs up as I lost my balls.

This is turning into an Oscar speech.

Thanks to Andrew & Sallie for your support and the wonderful times on the shrimper

Thanks also to Vanessa Townshend, professional make-up artist for her great work on me for the cover (www.vanessatownshend.co.uk) and John Reayner for getting me fit for life.

I wish to thank my wife, Mandy, whom without her support and motivation I would never have finished this book, given up excessive alcohol consumption and a list of other things as long as your arm that were basically killing me. All through our troubles, for five years she stood by me. Even when I was not the easiest person to stand by, she did. We fought this fight together. Sadly we were alone, but we won. We may be battered and bruised but we proved that when the chips are down, together we can beat anyone or anything. Our bond is too strong for anyone to break; I love you very much and thank you for everything.

Oh, and all peoples names from now on have been changed to protect their identity, except for John.

Now, shall we get on?

A MAN DERAILED

Introduction - The Why

First of all I would like to thank you for picking up my book and reading it. After all, why should you? You do not know me from Adam. You took a little leap of faith and I hope I live up to your expectations. For those of you who do know me, well thank you anyway, but let's face it, you had little choice and I know where you live. We shall say no more.

Yes, another book about someone's personal battle with mental illness, namely depression. I wanted to write something different to most other books I have read in the past about depression. Basically many of them did not seem to hold out much hope of ever having a fulfilling life. The problem being these books are usually typed out at times when that person truly believes that. I started this book, towards the end of a very serious bout of depression, nearly five years to be exact. If I wrote this four years ago, which would have been physically impossible, it would have sent you into a depressive episode too and that's not what I wanted to achieve. I wanted to show that there is hope and also to show non sufferers how they can help or indeed how their actions hurt the sufferer. Turning your back on someone that is suffering depression is like hitting a broken leg with a hammer: it bloody hurts and does more damage than the original problem.

I know exactly when my depression started: 7th

November 2003 at 2130 hours, and I know exactly where also, as you will see in due course. In that respect I am very lucky as there are thousands of people who have no idea why they are suffering with depression. Some have suffered all their lives without really understanding why. Others have suffered from circumstances that may be too horrific to remember or is it genetic? We just don't know. My thoughts go out to them.

The reason I am writing this book is to highlight the problems I faced while suffering from depression, anxiety disorder and post-traumatic stress. I am very sorry to disappoint you as I never hallucinated, was never sectioned or indeed carted away in a van with rubber walls, there are no wild and crazy stories about my excesses of booze and drugs. I never tried to kill myself, for this alone I am truly grateful. I guess you could say I have depression lite! My illness was free, most of the time, from psychotic tendencies. You didn't have to hide the sharp cutlery from me. I, from the outside was just an irrational miserable bastard who didn't want to socialise with any other human on the planet as I seemed to have lost the means of being able to connect.

Though this depression is bad, but not by any means the worse you can have, it also means it's a hell of a lot harder to get any decent treatment. To get anything done in this health service you have to either be slashing your own wrists or slashing someone else's. Basically until you are not acceptable to other people, then they will do something, eventually. However, if you aren't harming anyone else and running down the road naked in front of primary schools then you have to scream and shout till you are blue in the face to get anything done.

Once you get in the health system, they use a one size fits all policy when it comes to treatment. As you will see it's nonsense. While you live in a depressed state of mind 24 hours a day, you have to fight and battle for proper treatment. This is so hard to do.

So because I have only depression lite I do not put before you a diary of events, simply because it would be too boring. I mean, come on:

Day 1 Stayed in bed

Day 2 Stayed in bed

Day 3 Brushed teeth, stayed in bed (a good day)

Get the picture? So here we have chunks of my depressed life laid bare before you. It was hard to share the moments when I was at my lowest, it was hard to write, but I want others who go though the same things as I do to know you are not alone.

I want to share with you what happens when an employee from a very large company falls along the wayside, due to the company's own fault of course. Despite my depression and other problems I was left to totally fight for every piece of treatment I could get. It was a huge struggle and still is to this day. Throw into the melting pot a personal injury claim, crap managers, a crap union and therapists charging £100 per hour, you can then begin to imagine how frustrating a time this was.

If you are a sufferer of depression or any other illness that cannot be seen with the naked eye, you will understand how hard it is to try to explain what is wrong with you, why you are suffering and how someone can help you. Sometimes asking for help when you are your lowest ebb is the hardest thing to do. The shame of admitting you have failed in life, you feel worthless and so the vicious circle of depression starts.

For many of my close friends and family this will be the first time they will know the real truth of what happened to my wife and I after the crash. I guess some things may be hard to read or indeed shocking. The only thing I can say now is that it is written in past tense and as you will see I managed to beat many of my demons.

Anyway, put your feet up and stir your Prozac and coffee and let's try and make sense of it all . . .

Again, thank you for reading.

A MAN DERAILED

Chapter 1 - The How

Can you walk like a train driver?

Come on, you know what I mean. As he gets out of his driving cab he deliberately holds his rucksack over one shoulder making it look like it weighs 200 lbs and looks at the floor. As fast as his body allows he marches up the platform to the other end of the train, avoiding all eye contact with any other person on the platform. He usually looks like an old man carrying a bag of coal into a head-on wind. There is actually a perfectly good reason for this: it's to avoid a stupid conversation with passengers. As shown below:

Passenger: Excuse me! Is this the train to Cambridge?"

Driver: Do you mean this train here? The one with Cambridge written on it. The train on the platform marked "Train for Cambridge", the one with the automated message blaring out "THIS TRAIN IS FOR ALL STOPS TO CAMBRIDGE"?

Passenger : Erm, yes, is it the one?

Driver nods in disgust and moves on. Of course it can be quite daunting when travelling on the railway network and you aren't familiar with your surroundings, but as a train driver you tend to have this conversation at least a dozen times a day, it makes you turn into some xenophobic creature. Basically you spend all day on your own in the cab, a total solitary creature and then as soon as you get out of the cab you are bombarded with stupid questions. All you want to do when you pull your train into a terminus is to get to the other end as quick as possible, pull away and go home.

So you climb into your driving cab, turn all your lights off and wait for the right time to pull away again. You close the train doors, make your announcements and then the rest of the trip is just staring out of the window and watching the same old piece of scenery you have been driving past for years. It pays the bills.

I had become a train driver in 1998 and, though it was a work environment I was totally unprepared for, it turned out to be good for me. I had more time on my hands, despite the shift work, and a bloody good income. I went through all the training with some good people and we all worked together to get each other through the coursework and exams. Once you pass out the scariest thing is being given a train full of passengers to drive on your own for the very first time. All of a sudden you can't remember a thing. Where do I brake? Where am I stopping? You suddenly have total responsibility for hundreds of people's lives in the back of the train; it was a daunting time. Then after time you learn the train driver walk, avoid all humans, never work your break and get into the swing of things and settle down to the railway culture.

Friday 7th November 2003, the 2040 hours to Shoeburyness via Basildon was an important journey for me. It was the last time I ever climbed into a driver's cab and drove a train. I sat in my cab at Fenchurch Street, I could not wait to pull away. It was my last trip of the day: into Shoeburyness and then off work for 3 whole days, heaven. It was a pretty uneventful trip, as most journeys were. I was running on time, the train was full of drunk kids all going to Southend to enjoy some night life and drunk office workers coming home after a hard week behind the keyboard. Once you leave a station at night there is very little to see out of the cab window. You see other oncoming trains, stations in the distance and maybe the odd house, but mainly lit up railway track and loads and loads of gravel and ballast packed in underneath it.

Forty minutes into my journey I was contacted on the radio by the signalman. He was informing me that the train driver ahead had reported something strange happening and asked if I would inspect the line between the stations. This meant driving at 20 mph and looking at the line ahead. Also at night you have to get your guard upfront with you as two sets of eyes are better than one and I have to drive the train. I set the train in motion; we both stared out into the darkness looking down at the track that was lit up by the headlamps. As I got the train moving to 20 mph I leaned forward to see if I could see anything on the track, cursing as this was making my working day those few minutes longer. Then there was a huge explosion.

Explosions aren't like watching explosions in films

at the cinema. The noise is more of a thud. There were no flames but loads of sparks like fireworks exploding inches from my nose. Then there was nothing. The explosion had thrown me off my chair and into the centre of the cab. As my foot came off the "dead man's" pedal an alarm sounded and soon the brakes applied, bringing the train to a halt. The windscreen had shattered and there was a large hole in the body of the train. As I opened my eyes the cab was dark and all I could see was the imprint left on my retinas of the explosion. The left side of my head, face, neck and my left arm felt burnt, all the hair from my arms had gone or had melted. I felt the skin on my face tighten as if getting a whole summer's sunburn in one second.

My huge worry was my eyes. I did not know if it was dark or if my eyes were actually damaged. I could feel grit in my eyes. I didn't rub them as I knew there must be glass in there, I needed to get it out. The guard who was with me was in shock also but was further away from the explosion so thankfully did not have any apparent injuries. As I stood up I could not feel a thing through my whole body. I was not consciously doing anything. I was on auto pilot, part of my brain had switched off and it was as if I was watching myself do things from across the cab. My body had gone into deep shock. The next 20 minutes were somewhat of a blur. I had to contact the signaller, stop all train movements and request all power to the overhead cables had to be switched off. It soon became apparent what had happened. The overhead power cables had fallen down, crashed into the front of my train and earthed 25000 volts through my cab, inches from my face. If I had been travelling at line speed, 70 mph, I would be dead without a shadow of a doubt. Once we were told all the power had been switched off, the guard had to walk the passengers to the next station. This was crazy, as the previous station was around 500 yards behind us and the next station in front was 3 and half miles. This consisted of around 20 girls in high heels and miniskirts being made to walk on ballast for all that distance in the freezing cold. When they got there they wanted to string the guard up by his bollocks but it was not his fault, poor sod.

I was now left alone on a passenger train, in complete darkness. I had to secure the train the best I could and sit there and wait for managers and incident people from Railtrack to arrive. The train moaned and groaned as the air slowly seeped out of its suspension bags. As the time passed all the usual noises you hear on a train and take for granted ceased. I sat there in low level emergency lighting, no radio or mobile phone to contact the outside world. I had to sit there and wait. As I sat there I could feel the burns on my face. As I put my hand up to my face my beard felt weird: it had melted to my face. The hair on the side of my head had also melted and become like a lump of tar stuck to the side of it. The hair on my knuckles had gone, and the hair on my arms had also melted. My nose felt weird also. It was like there was a concrete bogey up my left nostril, I had to get it out, it felt sharp and was irritating. As

I rammed my finger up there, like you do, it felt like a hard piece of plastic had lodged up there. I tried to work it out as I scraped it out with my nail. I realised it was connected to me and my nasal hair had also melted to the inside of my nostril. The skin on my face felt so tight, it was so sore, a horrendous burning sensation. As the skin tightened I found it harder and harder to move my eye, my cheek and my lips. I kept waggling my jaw to loosen it but it would not work. I sat there, feeling a banging in my chest. The darkness seemed to close in on me, it was hard to see. I tried to squint but my left side of my face would not squint, it just failed to work.

All I wanted to do was to get home. As the managers turned up they just started to question me. The investigation officer from Rail track said to me in the fading light. "So how fast do you want me to say you were going?"

"I was going 20 miles per hour" I replied. I really could do with just getting out of here.

"Are you sure?"

"What do you mean am I sure? Of course I am."

"Well that's a big explosion for that speed. Are you sure? I mean we can find out from the black box you know, so if you want to change your story, now is the time." I looked at him with my one good eye and just wanted to punch his lights out. I mean at least in the films when you were being interrogated there was always the good cop and bad cop.

A MAN DERAILED

Where was the good cop? I felt as if I was in some murder enquiry. Of course I knew they could prove it, why would I lie? For the record, it turned out at the convenient closed inquiry they performed, I was not going at 20mph but 18mph so he can shove his assumptions up his arse. He then inquired if I was ok and then said do you want to go home or go to hospital? As I was not in any pain but in a complete state of numbness caused by the shock I chose the safest place I knew: home. In hindsight I should have gone to the hospital, but I was not thinking straight. Everything was like a weird dream and all I wanted to do was wake up in bed and say, "Phew, it was just a dream", roll over and go back to sleep.

I was escorted home by two members of staff. We got a cab and I sat in silence all the way home. As I opened the door my wife looked at me in shock horror. Her mouth was open and shouted, "Oh my God. Look, what happened to you?" I went upstairs to our bathroom and looked in the mirror. I could not believe what looked back at me. Half my face was brilliant red, the hair melted as I suspected to the side of my head, the rest of my hair was like a red afro. It had frazzled in the radiation and changed colour from mousey brown and grey to, well, ginger. The tightness of my face was no longer sore. I assumed with some after sun cream that it would soon heal or indeed peel. After a while talking to my wife it was obvious the tightness of the skin was making it hard for me to talk so we decided to go to bed. I closed my eyes, but the sleep would not come. My eyes kept flipping open, all I could see was the firework flash in and hear the weird thud of an explosion sound, over and over it played like a looped video tape. The strange thing was it was the silence after the crash that kept me awake. The period of time that I sat all alone on the train, waiting for something to happen. Waiting for someone to help me. It seemed to take forever. I was in the belly of a huge metal beast that was slowly dying. Its compressors had long stopped pumping air into huge suspension bags under the carriages. Slowly it leaked out, every inch the carriage dropped it made loud groaning noises. I could see nothing out of the window, just a faint outline of my reflection looking back at me lit up by the low powered emergency light. Finally I had heard the last groan and then there was silence. The silence was awful. It meant there was no one near me, no one coming and no one to help me. That feeling stayed with me throughout the coming years: the feeling of abandonment, that feeling of being completely alone.

I tossed and turned but could not sleep, I had to get up. I watched some TV; the pictures and the sound just washed over me without me really absorbing the program. I sat there on the sofa shaking, feeling sick, feeling alone. The only sound I made was the sniffling as the tears rolled down my face. I felt embarrassed: I was crying, I felt weak and I felt so alone.

A MAN DERAILED

Chapter 2 (alternative) - The Aftermath

The following morning after the crash I awoke from the little sleep I had had and tried to make sense of everything that had happened. I was lucky as it was a Saturday and my wife was at home so we were able to sit down and try to talk about what had happened. The whole memory seemed very surreal, all I was remembering were the flashes of sparks exploding across the windscreen of my train, the feeling on the right side of my face at it took some sort of electrical radiation burn and then nothing. One minute the whole cab was lit up with green sparks as far as the eye could see and then all the power went and I was left in complete darkness. It was like a crazy roller coaster ride: a burst of energy with extreme heat and light and then darkness and cold of the night. I do not know if I was unconscious. I know the train was emptied by my guard and I was left there for an eternity waiting until the management arrived. As for what I did or said I have no idea, I just seemed to go onto some sort of autopilot and my greatest desire was to get out of there and get to the only place I felt safe: that was home.

I could not eat breakfast the next morning; I had no feelings of hunger, just feelings of pure anxiety. I felt I had to be somewhere else or be doing something, anything, but I did not have a clue as to what. I stepped into the bathroom and turned on the shower. As the water started to steam I looked at my face in the mirror, my left hand side of my face was bright red like a severe sun burn. My eyelid did not move in time with the other eyelid and the surrounding area had no feeling whatsoever. I just assumed that it would be a like a sunburn and peel off over the next few days and everything would come back to some sort of normality. I stepped under my shower and the hot water splashed all over my head. I looked up to the shower head and then let the water engulf my face. I felt like I needed to wake up from a bad dream. The heat of the water was only apparent on the right side of my face; the left hand side was completely numb. It was a weird sensation. As I got out of the shower I started to re-examine my face in the mirror. As I looked I saw my sunken blackened eyes staring back at me. I was biting my lips trying to see if I had any feeling anywhere on the left side of my face. My eyelid, cheek, eyebrow all the way down to my jaw line were completely numb. I started to question myself about not going to the hospital directly after I left the incident. I know I should have but at the time I was on some sort of autopilot. All my instincts were saying to me, "Get home, just get home".

I booked an appointment with my GP and got an early appointment on the Monday morning. Going to the doctors was not something I did a lot of. I went into his room and explained what had happened. He looked at me for about 20 seconds umming and arrring and then asked if the redness was caused by the explosion. You have to remember half of my face was bright red and the other half was normal white skinned. I also only had half an eyebrow on the left hand side where I had to pick it off where it had melted and stuck to my skin. I looked at him and wanted to say, "No I just sunbathed on that side", but I resisted.

"You just have a partial Bells Palsy, nothing to worry about. If it has not cleared up in the next few weeks come back and we shall try some steroids, but these sort of things usually just sort themselves out." As usual I had gone to my GP and felt like I had wasted his time. Silly me, of course it was going to right itself, what the hell was I doing by going there and wasting his time?

I have to be completely honest now. I got home, sat down and the next 2 or 3 months are just a complete blur. I can tell you what started happening to me though. All of a sudden my house became my safe place. Each time I wanted to go out and do something I found it harder and harder to do so. If the door bell rang I would ignore it. I hated anyone coming into my sanctuary. The curtains were rarely opened; I kept the bad world out and my world separate to everyone and everything else. I started to watch 24 hour news coverage on cable TV. I watched as innocents in Iraq and Afghanistan were blown up on a daily basis. Keeping the rest of the world out of my house was the right thing to do, just look at what was happening to it. War seemed to dominate everything on the news. The more I watched the more sensitive I became to it. I started to feel as if it was happening just down the road, maybe in the next street. The gaps in-between leaving the house got bigger and bigger to the point where it could be counted in months and not days, or indeed weeks. I seemed to have only 2 mood settings: depressed and angry. When I was depressed I felt as if I was in a fog, I could not think straight, I did not eat, I hated myself as I felt weak. I used to deal with bad situations on a daily basis in my last job. Why the hell has one explosion affected me in this way? I had failed. I was no longer a strong man. What was the point of going on like this? I would be better off dead. Who wants a failure like this? When I was angry, my thoughts were clear. I could focus on something and argue till I was blue in the face, but I couldn't give up.

I had to argue and fight till I won or whoever else had backed down. I was angry against my employers for letting this happen to me, I was angry against the whole world for letting me go through all this on my own. Of course I was not alone, I had my wife for support and she did a great job, but she had to work; we still had a mortgage and bills to pay. She still had to commute up to London every day to keep the money coming in. Those were the hardest times. I was alone for 10 hours plus a day and slowly over time my thoughts and actions became darker and darker. A big black dog had taken control of every part of my brain. It sat with me 24/7. It would never leave me alone; I sat there every day wanting it to go but doing nothing about it. I was too tired from the lack of sleep and lack of food. I did not think I was worthy enough to tell anyone how I felt. I hated myself too much to want to be better. I didn't deserve it. Surely there were others who should have my quality of life I dreamt of. I was being punished. I do not know what for, but I must be, how else can you explain this? I wanted to never wake up in the morning, but this didn't happen purely because I did not sleep. I would fall asleep during the daytime. My head would fall forward as I sat in front of the television with the news showing death and destruction blaring in front of me. My take on life was completely warped. I did not trust anyone, I did not want to see anyone. My paralysed face made me feel ugly, the numbness felt like it had grown even bigger, just like I had had a dentist's anaesthetic. It was as if a huge growth was forming on the side of my mouth. I could see but no one else seemed to be able to, maybe they were just humoring me, who knows?

My face also had some scars where I would cut myself shaving. In the end I would give up shaving at all and allowed the beard to catch up with the rest of my already grown goatee. I felt as if my appearance had changed beyond all recognition. I hated the mirrors and would never look at them as I walked past them. I hated my reflection; all I saw looking back at me was a miserable, scruffy man who seemed to have lost his soul. His eyes were sunken and black. It was not me, it could not be. I never looked like this. Someone had stolen my smile. Don't get me wrong, I was never the life and soul of the party but I did smile now and then. This creature, I observed, looked as if he had never smiled in his life. Even worse, he looked like he was never going to either. My black dog had taken hold of me, I had full blown depression. I was ashamed to admit it. Who the hell am I going to tell? Slowly, as each day went past, I was to become more and more engulfed in the darkness of my thoughts.

A MAN DERAILED

Chapter 3 - So! You Think You Have Depression, Do You?

Well, so you have read how I came to have my very own black dog to keep me company. No matter what time of day it was or indeed is, he would always be close by. So what happens when you get your own black dog? Well, you have depressive symptoms, you constantly feel low and the bastard illness will not let you function normally no matter what you do or when you do it. Here is what should happen . . .

Step 1: Get depression. Now you can do this by numerous ways. If you are lucky you won't have to do anything at all and some bastard will cause it for you. This can be done by taking drugs, being abused, post-traumatic stress (that's my fav) or maybe an illness. It could be a million and one reasons why you get it, so don't worry, the chances are good.

Step 2: Do not be embarrassed or feel weak. You know you have it so you must go and get help and hit the black dog smack bang in the middle of the nose, making him whelp out loud and run off with his tail between his legs. Remember, everyone loves a depressed person.

Step 3: Go to the doctor. Your conversation with your GP should go like this: "Well Mr. Smith, what can I do for you?"

"I have felt very low lately, I can't concentrate or focus on my work, my wife thinks I am miserable all the time, I just cannot fathom it out" is one of the millions of replies you could give.

"I feel your pain Mr. Smith. This is a job for Super Psych and Therapo the depression busting duo," he replies and presses the psycho lamp which beams a light spelling CBT onto the clouds above.

Step 4: Super Psych sees you, almost immediately. You walk right into his office, barely touching the floor of the waiting room. He tells you all you need to know about your problems and gives you literature to show your family and friends. This is to create a completely supportive environment to help you heal and make a full recovery. He gives you the magic tablets which take away all your cares, allow you to eat properly and have 8 hours of natural sleep a day without any side effects. He needs to see you in a few months, as others are calling on his amazing powers. He then arranges a course of CBT with his sidekick, Therapo.

Step 5: You see Therapo almost weekly and over the few weeks you attend you have challenged all those nasty negative thoughts and feelings, you have started running marathons again and you play the violin like a pro.

Step 6: You are weaned off the tablets and Super Psych sees you for the last time. You are stronger, faster and more positive than an electric pylon. God bless the system. All you need to do now is write the book on your experiences and sell it to a large publishing house. Apparently people like to read that sort thing.

Well there you go, six easy steps to being cured. "Well hang on!!!" you ask, "If it was that easy and simple why are their sooooo many people suffering with depression?" Well, my dear reader, what you have just read is what should happen. In the real world it is quite different. Let's look and see what really goes on.

Step 1: Well that pretty much remains the same. If you are going to suffer with depression then it is going to happen. Sorry.

Step 2: Most of the time, most people who suffer with depression will not understand what is happening to them and would be too ashamed and embarrassed to ask a GP for fear they would not be taken seriously. They would feel weak and that they have failed in life. Over time they would feel they aren't worthy of any help, they feel no one will understand and deteriorate to the point where they would feel they are a liability and most people would be better off if they were dead. It is not until most sufferers get to this point that anyone will take you seriously or indeed want to help. If you feel these symptoms: feelings of hopelessness, inadequacy, anxiety, self-hatred, negativity, an inability to enjoy things which were once pleasurable in life, guilt, agitation, weight loss or weight gain, loss of energy or motivation, loss of sex-drive, disturbed sleep, poor concentration, indecisiveness, irritability, anger, social withdrawal, unexplained aches and pains, self-harm, recurring thoughts of death or suicide, then get down to the doctors. It is important to get into the system. If you feel you need help, I am sorry to say also, it is a system. A slow moving conveyor belt with the weird and wonderful moving along slowly in the void called the National Health System. It stinks, but ho hum, what you going to do? Unless you got a few grand lying around then I am afraid it is definitely the waiting game for you. However, you have to complete step three to start this process.

Step 3: The GP visit. Let's face it, we are incredibly lucky in this country to have a health system that is completely free to us. There are countries where people have died out of poverty, just because they cannot afford to pay for medical bills, millions of them, it's a disgrace. So we should be very proud of a system with amazing doctors, nurses and consultants. Thousands of lives have been saved in our NHS and thousands have a better way of life because of it. So why is the mental health system so crap? Mental health needs to be taken more seriously, but it isn't. WHY?

So here goes your first conversation with a health professional, usually your GP. Here is how it goes:

"Well Mr. Smith, what can I do for you?"

"I have felt very low lately. I cannot concentrate or focus on my work, my wife thinks I am miserable all the time, I just cannot fathom it out" is one of the millions of replies you could give again.

A MAN DERAILED

"Feeling a bit cheesed off are we?" he replies.

"Cheesed off?" Your back is up.

"Yes, fed up, got the blues? Awww bless." He continues playing solitaire on his computer.

"Well, if you mean I would like to walk into McDonald's and blow every fucking bastard in there away, then jump under a passing bus, then yes I am fucking cheesed off" he then replies.

"Well what do you want me to do about it?" Let's face it, if you knew what to do you would not be there would you? Now refrain from violence ok? It's hard getting onto another surgery's books when you have killed a doctor, especially in this day and age. It takes 14 or so years to train up a new one and you will spend that in jail. So take some deep breaths and say the four hardest words in the world it is to say when you have depression.

"Can you help me?" Well five if you are polite and say please.

He sits back in his chair and looks at his watch as your 3 minutes are almost coming to an end. "Ok," he smiles, "how about some drugs?" Don't worry, he is not going to get a bong out with you both sitting there for hours putting the world to rights while devouring six bargain buckets of KFC. He means:

ANNOUNCER: LET'S PLAY THE ANTIDEPRESSANTS GAME. *QUEUE MUSIC AND FLASHING LIGHTS . . .*

DOCTOR : Welcome ladies and gentlemen, and welcome to the antidepressant game. With me today we have Mr. Smith.

MR SMITH : Hi.

DOCTOR : So, you have bad sleep, you do not eat properly, you want to kill everyone that smiles, you have no appetite for sex, you drink to excess and you have severe anxiety attacks and very bad dreams.

MR SMITH : Erm yes, yes I do.

CROWD : AWWWWWWWWWWWWW

DOCTOR : Well Mr. Smith, as you can see we have the wheel of madness behind separated into 8 sections. Let's hear what's in each section.

Announcer: In one . . . we have a new antidepressant that makes you constipated and gives you severe migraines.

In two . . . Pull yourself together . . . you will feel much better when you are back at work.

In three . . . Counselling . . . You have to slit at least one wrist before we give you this one, so keep your fingers crossed.

In four . . . A psychiatrist . . . you must be joking . . . Not in a million years . . . We won't have any money left for the Christmas tree decs.

In five . . . An old antidepressant that gives you the

shits and stops you from driving your car. It's cheap, cheerful and addictive.

In six . . . A sick note for a fortnight and see how things go. Hopefully you will get another doctor next visit.

In seven . . . I haven't got a fucking clue. So I shall make you feel like you are wasting my time.

In eight . . . It's the doc's star prize . . . Yes, a referral for real ongoing treatment. NO WAY.

DOCTOR : So my little nutcase, let's spin the wheel.

THE CROWD GO WILD.

It may as well be like this. After all, anything your doctor does will start with the magical words that us depressives cannot stand. "Right, OK. Let's try . . ." If you were lying in bed with a broken arm or leg and the consultant stood next to you and said, "Right, OK. Let's try paracetamol" you would get off the bed and run like hell, or limp like hell. The problem is you can see a broken leg or arm. You can see it on the x-ray machine and it lights up magically on the screen and they know exactly what to do. With depression there is nothing but symptoms. They cannot see them, only in your mood and maybe they will learn from what you tell them. The problem also is that you never ever say what you want when you are in there. You always wish you had said this or that but you were pushed out of the door with a prescription for whatever he gave you and that's the end of that.

It usually ends with the words, "Try these for 3 months and come back to me and let me know how you are getting on." You will not challenge this because he is a doctor and knows best. I am sad to say this is not the case.

So you go back three months later and you say "I am still depressed, can you help me?" In theory you will then move down the conveyor belt to step 4.

Step 4: I am afraid Super Psych is not all he is cracked up to be either. You will have to wait months for an assessment. This will usually last one hour. The first 15 minutes you spend in the waiting room as he is running late, and the last 15 minutes he is rushing you out of the room as he wants to get back on time with his schedule. Who can blame him? It's not like you are the queen or anything. So you are sitting in a room full of people with severe mental health problems, which is fun. These are usually the times when you wonder if you should be sitting there or not. The room is not just filled with other depression sufferers, it has all sorts. When I first went to my NHS assessment I waited 45 minutes to go in. During that time I watched some incredibly ill people come and go. I watched as the receptionists booked people in through their bulletproof windows.

"Just take a seat sir and you will be called in shortly."

"Fuck off you bastard." shouts a huge bald man in shorts and a vest. It was December and no, it was not me.

"That's right, take a seat" the receptionist would reply.

All the receptionists would talk nice and slow and clear.

"Heeeeeeellllllllooooooooooooooo, hoooooooooooooooooow caaaaaaaaaaaaaaaaaan IIIIIIIIIIIIIIIIIIIIIIIIIIIIIIIIIIIIIIIIIIIIII Heeeeeeeeelllllpppp Youuuuuuuu?"

"I have an appointment at 10am with Doctor Patel."

"OOOOOOOOOOOOOOOOOOOOKKKKKKKKKKKKK KKKK, whaaaaaaaaaaaaaaaaaaaaaaaaaat'sssssssssss youuuuuuuuuuuuuuuuuuuuuurrrr naaaaaaaaaaaaaaaaaammmmeee ppppppooooooooollllllllleeeeeeaaaaaaaasssssssssse ?" she would say through the holes in the glass.

It was very sweet and they all seemed to have developed calming voices. I reckon they could present children's programs or do voice-overs. I then get called into a room by Doctor Patel who is a young lady fresh out of medical school and English is not quite her first language. Now, before you shout the racist card at me, I have to say I really appreciate the immigrant population who have come here to improve their own lives and indeed ours by filling the gaps in the health system. I do however believe that a psychiatrist should have a good standard of English as it is an illness that can only be analysed etc. etc. by talking alone. You cannot x-ray depression. So no offence, but this is how part of my assessment went.

After asking me 30 questions about my life in general and my history she then asked me why I am there. I explained that I may have post-traumatic stress, anxiety problems and indeed depression due to an incident that happened when I was driving my train. I then went into great detail about the explosion and all the other bits that you should know about as you were supposed to have read that bit at the beginning. She nodded at all my points I gave and things went on smoothly. She then got up and said, "I will be back in a minute." So off she went, carrying my file and a pen. Five minutes later she came back:

Doctor: So Mr. Holmes, this car crash, when did it happen exactly?

Me: It was a train crash, not a car crash.

Doctor: Your car was hit by a train?

Me: No, I was driving the train. That's what I do, I am a train driver.

Doctor: So where was your car when this happened?

Me: It was in the bloody car park at work.

Doctor: WOW, so your train went into the car park

and hit your car?

Me: My car was nowhere near it. I was in a train, I did not hit a car, I was hit by electric cables that earthed through my cab.

Doctor: So you were driving a cab?

Me: NO, A TRAIN, I WAS DRIVING A BLOODY TRAIN.

Doctor: Please calm down Mr. Holmes, you must be more clear.

Me: "My train was moving and the electric that powers the train from an overhead cable," pointing above my head, God knows why, "came down and sent electricity through my train and then caused an explosion which exploded in my face causing a head injury and post-traumatic stress symptoms."

Doctor: "Please wait, I will come back."

Again she left for 5 minutes, with my file and a pen. She came back, sat down with a prescription for an antidepressant no less.

Doctor: "OK, these will help with your symptoms, take them for 3 months and then come back and let us know how you are getting on."

Me: "So these will help my depression?"

Doctor: "Oh, so you have depression also?"

Me: "Well, shouldn't you be telling me?"

Doctor: "Well, you said you had post-traumatic stress and you can have that as well with depression, so yes, you can have that also."

Me: "Gee thanks."

I could have said anything really and they would have done exactly the same thing. Given me drugs for three months, then asked me to come back. If I was better, hey presto I am cured, if I feel ill still they just adjust the dose up or down and that's it. They will do anything not to give you therapy. If you do get put on the list the chances are by the time you get to the date you will either be better or dead, it takes ages.

Step 4 doesn't always go this smoothly. Sometimes I am sure it can be much worse. The problem is when you go back for the second appointment and tell them that the drugs they have prescribed to you aren't working or they have some severe side effects, they look at you as if you have just slapped them in the face. After all, what you are saying to them is that they were wrong. The drugs they supplied didn't work and they got it wrong. The thing is they didn't get it wrong as much as they have not got a clue. So when they say, "OK let's try these for three months and see how it goes," that is what they really mean. So for three months you are a guinea pig popping pills praying they help you sleep. So if they don't work then all that happens is they increase the dose. So you start to constipate and dehydrate a bit more, but feel worse. All they say in response to that is, "Oh, you have to give

them time. They need to get into your system."
The fact that I am shitting concrete bricks once a week and my lips are as dry as cornflakes tells me it's in my system well and truly. So after realizing that just pumping drugs into you won't work, they then refer you to therapy. So we hop skip and jump to step 5.

Step 5: You will now go and see a therapist. You sit down and talk and work things through. It can be a huge relief to just sit down in a room with someone who is going to just listen and not actually judge you. They will then talk about steps on how to move forward and how to gain control back from the black dog. Let's face it, depression controls you whether you like it or not and here we learn the skills of how to beat it away and gain some quality of life back. Sometimes we win and sometimes we lose, but it helps us not give up. It's hard, but in my opinion the therapist is the most important person, other than you, who can actually make a difference.

Step 6: Well this takes a long time to come. Some people are on meds for life and have ongoing treatment for years. There is no real rule on when you are cured or, indeed, if you are cured. It is widely accepted that once you have bouts of depression you can have them over and over again or it may never happen again. If you do come out the other side, make sure you don't take your mental health for granted and learn your lessons. After all, no one else will tell you.

Get on the conveyor belt and good luck.

Chapter 4 - You Will Feel a Prick

It became clear after a short period of time that the injury to my face was not going to go away as quickly as I got it. From my eyebrow down to my jaw line was completely numb and very difficult to move. Even when I drink a cup of tea to this day I leave drips of tea on the outside of the mug where my bottom lip cannot seem to get in the right place. I mean, in the scheme of things, it's not a huge problem but it's like a constant reminder of what happened in the past. No one was particularly sympathetic about the injury, after all it didn't leave loads of scarring and I didn't have bits of me dropping off. If I didn't speak or try to smile, which is not hard to do when you are depressed, you would not even know I had it. So this meant that every medical exam I had for the paralysis started with, "Oh well, it doesn't look that bad does it?"

"Well as long as it doesn't fucking bother you then, everything is alright." I would reply in my usual charming way. The fact it bothered me was neither here nor there as far as they were concerned and this did not help me in my ever decreasing mental state. As everyone tried to pretend it wasn't there, it made me feel as if I was stupid to even mention it. I mean what the hell was I playing at? A third of my face did not have any feeling in it and it could not function properly and there I was being a big baby and trying to sort it out. I don't know, what the hell was I thinking? The problem was it was smack bang on my face, I saw it every day in the mirror until I stopped looking in the mirror. I grew a full beard in the hope that it would stop me from noticing, but it just did not work. I just had a lop-sided beard and loads of grey in it, which also started making me think of my own mortality. I guess it's sort of like a midlife crisis; grey hair does that to you. So here I was with a grey beard, a lop-sided mouth, I had severe depression, anger management problems and severe anxiety problems. Not the sort of bloke you wanted to prop a bar up with I can tell you.

After some pestering, I got my GP to actually do his job and got referred to a neurologist. After some negotiating it was finally agreed to be paid privately by my company and off I went up to the local private hospital to be examined. My consultant was a very glamorous Middle Eastern lady, made up to the nines with the usual white coat and stethoscope dangling from her neck.

"Mr Holmes, you are quite obese!"

"Thank you, I didn't realise, I thought I was just big boned. Does it have a relevance to why my face is not working?"

"No, I am just making general observations, it's what I must do." She replied.

"Can I do that as well?" I growled back.

"Erm shall we continue?"

Through my illness, and I am sure it will happen in the future, every report that was ever written about me started with, "Mr Holmes is obese." Hey lets really fuck up my self esteem and put it all in black and white for all to see. Why not take some fucking pictures while you are at it and post them on the web; go on, really humiliate me. It's a shame the consultants do not spend as much time trying to make things right as they do trying to pad out their reports so it looks like it's worth the vast sums of money they are being paid for it.

She took my blood pressure and did lots of poking around my face. She would take a paperclip and unravel it, then dig it into various parts of my face and I had to tell her if I felt it. One thing I cannot stand, and that is touching my actual eyeballs. If I ever had to wear contact lenses I just would not be able to do it. As the finger with the lens would get nearer and nearer to my eye I would lean backwards trying to get further and further away. So when she decided to roll some cotton wool up into a point and then try to poke me in both eyes to see if I could feel it, the atmosphere got a little tense to say the least.

"You don't actually have to touch my right eye, that's fine." She ignored me and slowly pushed the white pointy cotton wool closer to my right eye. My natural reaction was to lean back and as I did she grabbed my head to stop my motion. I stared right at the gnarly point and she jabbed it into my eye. I immediately blinked and streams of tears poured down my cheek. "So, you felt that, yes?"

A MAN DERAILED

I nodded my head. I gave in and allowed her to do the same with the other eye. It was weird, I could see the tip heading towards me, I wanted to blink, but I held firm and waited for the same feeling as the right eye. There was nothing. She prodded it again and I didn't flinch. After another 5 minutes of prodding she said, "We need to test the nerves in your head. I will arrange for you to go to the hospital to have the cranial nerves tested to see if there is a break in them."

I got sent home and waited for the appointment to come through in the post. I have to be honest, I had no idea what these tests would consist of. I just assumed it meant a few wires with sensors on being stuck to my head which monitor my brain waves or something along those lines. Oh I was so wrong.

Ok, picture this if you will. I have a natural fear of needles, nothing to do with the crash, I have always had it. If I have to give blood or have any injection I almost faint, especially if I see the needle going in. I don't feel the same if it goes in someone else, just me. Nothing exciting about that I suppose and I think quite a natural fear to have. My new fear was now electricity. I don't mean plug sockets in the wall, I don't scream every time I see shaver socket, I mean sparks and sounds that electricity can give off. I seemed to have become very sensitive to power cables, especially in the wet and winter months. So this made me a great candidate to have 4 needles pushed in my head and then send an electric current in to my head to see what muscles constricted and what muscles did not. Hey, they were so nice about it. They gave me a big bit of rubber to bite on to so I did not bite my tongue off; how sweet. What the hell was wrong with these morons? I felt like I was in a scene from One Flew Over the Cuckoo's Nest. At least they didn't strap me down. If I knew what was going to happen and protested, I would not have put it past them.

So here I am sitting on a table with my feet off the ground in some dingy Portakabin and the rear of the hospital. I guess they did this there as no one can hear you scream from there. The needles were shown to me by the doctor. They were sitting there in a dish that you usually see gallstones being dropped into during an operation. In front of me was what I now know to be some sort of generator that sent the electricity down the needles via some wiring into my face. It was so old. In fact it had rust on the corners of it and various dials to increase or decrease the voltage. It would not have looked out of place in a 1950s sci-fi film. The thing I will never forget was the size of the needles: they were at least 4 inches long; that's ten centimetres for you younger readers and they were thick. I did query the thickness of the needle and was told not to worry as they were only going to be pushed into the skin at various points and no deeper than that. That was a relief because they were going to stick them into my head.

Either side of me there is a nurse with a clipboard. Their job is to see how I react once the surge of electricity flows through my head. I had a sneaky feeling I could have told them all this in advance and avoided all this, but who was I to ruin all their fun? First they were going to test my fully functioning side of my face. I told them it worked completely well but they needed to test it so they can compare my non functioning side. The doctor picks up the dish of needles and leans forwards. Holding the first needle between his first finger and his thumb, he leans forward saying, "This will be the earth." and pushed it into the base of my chin, through my beard. I felt the bluntness of the needle. It did not pierce my skin but seemed to bludgeon its way though. Basically it bloody hurt. Then he put another three needles of the exact same size into my right eyebrow, cheek and then my jaw line. The needles stuck out of my head and I could feel them tugging on my skin. Then I felt a warm liquid sensation, oh good I was bleeding. The nurse grabbed swabs of some sort with her latex covered hand and started to mop up my blood before it stained my tee shirt. Then one by one the doctor connected the needles to red wires with crocodile clips, making sure he put the right wire to the correct needle. The extra weight of the clips and wire made the needles tug even more on my face and it became extremely uncomfortable.

"Ok Mr Holmes, I am going to send three bursts of electricity through so make sure you are biting on the rubber bung please. Are you ready?" Have you ever tried to answer someone while biting down on a rubber bung? I just nodded. Then it hit me. The first burst was like a huge slap around the face, followed by my muscles constricting so much I thought my jaw was being pulled up to my forehead. As I flinched the needles pulled more and I could feel more blood pouring down my face. It was a good ten seconds before I could get my breath. My jaw ached as my teeth tried to slice the rubber bung in half; thank God I had it. If my tongue was there it would definitely have been sliced off.

"OK Mr Holmes, here we go again." Before I had a chance to say,

"Touch that dial and I will fucking kill you," the second wave of electricity surged through my head. It was weird and painful. My face was trying to do things that I had no control over, my anxiety levels went through the roof and I pulled the needles out. The nurses, who were scribbling things down on their clipboards, put the boards down and tried to stop me. "What the fuck are you doing?" I shouted, "Get them out of me, get them out now." They pulled the remaining needles out and got me some water and tried to calm me down. The doctor was totally unsympathetic. "How can we do our job if we cannot run our tests?" I just looked at him and wanted to jam the needles in him and give him a blast, see how he would like it.

What I soon learned from this was that a neurologist is only interested in the physical problem at hand; he doesn't see the whole picture. I do not know why, it was all in my file, but they choose not to read it. I was in a crash and damaged by electricity and have an irrational fear of electricity. I also have a severe mental problem of depression, but that just did not seem to matter. His bedside manner left a lot to be desired and I could not get out of there quick enough.

After about ten minutes, I agreed to let him do it one more time on my numb side. Again he inserted the earth in the chin which I felt and then the same needles in the same places only on the left side of my face. I did not feel a thing, but again blood oozed down my face and was kindly mopped up by the nurses. Like Dr Frankenstein, he sent his electricity through my head. Again my whole jaw contracted and so did my eyelids but the pain was a lot less. For some reason I instinctively stood upright, ripping the needles from my face. Again I wanted to head for the exit.

"Wait, wait, come on Mr Holmes, sit down and have a drink of water before you leave." They did this as they did not want me to walk back out in to the waiting room covered in blood and obviously distressed. It took me ages to calm down. Once my blood flow had been stemmed and I was cleaned up I left. I had not got a clue what they wrote down or what their findings were. All I knew was I had to get home. They were exactly the same feelings I had on the night of the crash itself. Home was where I wanted to be as it felt safe. Little did I know that years later home would seem like a jail cell and all I dreamt of was trying to escape it.

The big mistake I made that day was that I drove there. This meant I had to drive back home. I got in my car and wound the window down. The parking in our local hospital is a nightmare. As soon as I got in my car there was already another car waiting for me to get out. I needed to sit there and collect my thoughts, my head was banging away and my neck and face on the right side felt like it had been lifting heavy eights and seemed to be strained. My left eye socket ached and I had to squint to see properly; it was awful. Then someone pressed their car horn for me to move. I didn't even look, I just sat there. I didn't care as I was not ready to move. I held my face in my hands and rubbed it hoping to make it feel easier, but my headache got stronger and stronger as if pressure was building up inside. I needed to lie down.

They beeped their horn again, I got out. Behind me was a very old man and I assume his wife in a small car behind. I stared at them and shouted, "Fuck off, I am not moving." I saw the fear in their eyes as he slammed the gear stick into reverse and pulled away. I was not proud of myself but I needed to just be left alone. I also realised why they looked so scared: some of the holes were leaking again and I had streams of blood down my face. I needed to get home. I turned the engine on and left the car park. I drove as if looking through a snow storm. I had to squint, the sun was too bright and my headache seemed to be turning into a migraine. Thankfully it was a quiet time of day as far as the roads were concerned and I got home quite quickly. I parked and walked into my house. I washed my face in the bathroom and dried it, making sure the bleeding had stopped, and then laid on my bed. Closing my eyes eased the headache but each time I closed my eyes I saw the sparks from the crash. This had brought it all back to me and I felt as raw and vulnerable as I did from the first day of the crash. I didn't leave the bed for several days.

Two weeks later I got a letter confirming I had damaged two cranial nerves. Basically it said there was no surgical procedure that could help and it may well heal itself over time. In other words there was nothing they could do; I would just have to live with it. Over time, small patches of my face got feeling and movement back. Now it looks normal but there are some numb patches. You can usually spot them as they are the bits I cut when shaving; just a little reminder I keep just to remind me of the crash, in case I forget you understand.

Chapter 5 -The Counselor

After months and months of being left to rot and fester in my cage I now called home, I got a phone call out of the blue. It was a particularly bad day for me, I was extremely low and feeling like no one cared and all the 101 other negative feelings I usually let rule my life. The phone kept ringing and I held it in my hand with the little screen flashing with a local number. I took a deep breath and decided to answer it before the anxiety and fear took over. I pressed the accept call button and then there was a voice at the other end. Of course there was a voice, I hear you saying, but it was quite a voice. She sounded as if she had just spent the morning riding ponies with her three children and then was on her way to read the shipping forecasts on Radio 4. She certainly didn't sound local.

"Oh hello, Paul, my name is Martha. I have been asked by ICAS to arrange an appointment with you with a view of some counselling for you." Her voice was quite something; it conjured up loads and loads of different pictures in my head, her sitting there in her riding britches and boots wielding a crop in her hand saying, "Get better or I will whip your bottom. Now beg for sugar cubes." Well I was pretty fucked up in the head so what do you expect? We arranged an appointment and she gave me directions of where to go, it was going to be at her house, and we said our goodbyes.

All of a sudden I was on the conveyor belt of

treatment for my black dog. How bizarre it would come from some frightfully posh woman who lived in what I thought was some country mansion out of town. This would mean not only would I have to meet someone new but also drive somewhere and go into new surroundings. It was all quite scary really. As usual the appointment was for about a month ahead so my brain played every single scenario possible and all of them would be bad. I would think how I would break down my car on the way and be trapped in a field with nothing but cornfields and scarecrows. I would be found days later in my car surviving on grass and water from my windscreen washers. Then I believed she was part of my work place and was hired to investigate me to see if I was actually telling the truth. I believed they thought I was faking the whole thing and sooner or later I would be dragged kicking and screaming to a train drivers cab and made to drive it with 800 people on board.

These soon encroached into my dreams for the few hours I slept. As I lay there I would be dreaming the most ridiculous scenarios but they felt so real. The dream that stayed with me, even to this day, is the following. I pull away from a station and all is well. Soon I come to the point where I must apply the brakes for the next station and the handle comes off in my hand. The train speeds up and rattles along at great speed. I am pushing buttons, trying to take my keys out of the computerised console. As I look out of the screen we fly off the tracks over the bridge in town and derail, causing the train to fly off the bridge and land on the pedestrianised high street. We continue at a rate of knots, people jumping out of my way and just as I was about to crash into the Ann Summers shop I always wake up. I wake up with a full start, covered in sweat. It feels so real and, even when I dream it now, it feels like it is actually happening. I have always wondered what happens when I crash the train into the Ann Summers shop. I try to stay asleep but I never can, the point of impact at the glass in the front is always too scary. Perhaps I crashed through the glass and wake up covered in red warm liquid only to be told, "Don't worry son, its only strawberry lubricant, you'll make it."

I knew I had to talk about these dreams, minus the strawberry lubricant of course, and I needed to find a way of stopping the rot and my decline into a worse depressive state.

The day of the appointment came. The previous night I was so anxious I could not sleep. I laid there staring at the ceiling; my brain not switching off, it was as if it was scared to go, as it would rid it of this parasite that controlled me. It was scared and so was I. Luckily enough it was an early morning appointment which meant not having the whole day to talk myself out of going. Even if she is a spy for the other side I will just go and tell the truth, I have nothing to hide. The problem was, the more I thought this of her the more I wanted to clam up and not say a word. She must have some sort of ulterior motive. I had been off work now for almost six months, no one from my place of employment had contacted me and I did not have a clue if I was going to be sacked or helped. Maybe I would find out more here.

My GPS system consisted off some badly scrawled directions on the back of a phone bill and amazingly I got there avoiding the scarecrows and corn of which there was none. She lived in what looked like an ex council house on the edge of town, it was respectable but not many horse boxes on the back of Range Rovers were parked along the street. I pulled up and parked my car and was just relieved that I actually got there in one piece. The sweat rolled down my back and my heart raced. As I drove along each street felt as it if were six lanes in each direction and for some reason I totally did not have a clue where I was going as I had lost all my confidence in driving. So after the initial shock, came relief that I did get there.

I pressed the door bell and through the frosted glass I could see a figure approach. As she opened the door two cats ran out, startling me, and then Martha stood in front of me with a big smile and with her booming posh voice she welcomed me in. She was very short, quite round and had huge glasses on with short red hair that had been styled in a way that most middle aged women seem to have. She ushered me into her sitting room and I sat on a sofa. She sat on the single seat in front of me, her feet not touching the carpet. As we started to talk and she asked me why I was there, a collection of cats started to converge on me. One on my lap then two on the headrest of the sofa. Then a tabby who decided that my legs made excellent scratching posts. "Fuck" I shouted as the claws went through my trousers and into my skin. As I did so all the cats scattered and hid in various nooks and crannies around the room.

"Paul, I am so sorry, do you mind cats? I can get them out of the room if you wish?"

"No, I love cats," I replied. "I didn't expect them to dig their claws into my leg, it hurt. I am sorry; I didn't mean to scare them." As we started the session, minus the cats, we talked about the crash and my feelings to those responsible. What was quite apparent was my anger for what had happened. I was just not angry about what happened, but I really hated those responsible and how they had just left me to hang out to dry all alone with no help to try and get well.

"Perhaps they are just giving you space so you can start to get well again. Perhaps they feel any contact will be seen as pressure to return to work?" she would say, trying to make sense of it all.

"Are you telling me that a phone call asking me how I am is pressurising me to go back to work?" I angrily replied. I started to believe she was on their side.

"No of course not, I am sure they have their reasons though."

"Yes they do," I grunted. "They don't give a shit and they are more pissed off they have to cover my work than they are about what happened."

A MAN DERAILED

"No Paul, I am sure they have handled this badly, but I am sure they care."

"Actions speak louder than words, and I have had neither," I replied angrily. It was apparent the angrier I got the clearer I saw everything. At least from what I believed. Why would no one contact me from my employers to ask how I am? If I was a manager of someone I would ring them. I would say things like, "What do you need to get better," or "If there is anything you need just ring." The problem is, I never got those calls and here was a woman trying to convince me that they cared. This was five months after the crash and I had not heard a thing from them, so make of it what you will, but I was pretty pissed off. Martha sensed this and decided to talk about channeling my energies into other things other than being angry all the time.

At the end of the session, as we did with the following five sessions, we performed an incredibly weird ritual. Now it was not intended to be weird, it just kind of turned out that way. She came over to me and said, "Paul, I want you to get comfortable, place your feet on this foot stall and rest your head back on the sofa and close your eyes. " I did as requested and sunk myself into the spongy sofa and tried to relax. The minute my feet went onto the foot rest two cats would jump on my lap and make themselves comfortable as well. I did not mind this; as they settled and started purring it was really quite relaxing. Then she would turn on her CD player and start to play some relaxing music. It sounded like guitars and synthesizers playing a slow melodic tune and in the background was the sound of whale calls and water. With my eyes closed the relaxation time began. She would start to talk and I had to follow her every word.

"Okay, I want you to be somewhere where you feel so relaxed. If it could be anywhere in the world, where would it be?"

"Fistral Beach, in Cornwall" I slowly replied in my trance like state. "Ahhhh Cornwall, so beautiful. I want you to imagine walking along that beach now. Feel the sunshine warming the skin of your face and arms. Feel the winds caressing you and cooling you, feel the sea spray in the winds on your face. Imagine the sand under your feet, so soft. I want you to feel all these feelings and see them in your mind. Imagine you are really there, walk out to the sea and feel the water lash up against your feet and ankles, feel calm, feel good and reeeeeeeeeeeeeellllllaaaaaaaaaaaaaaaaaaaaaaaa aaaaaaaaaaaaaaaaax. I want you to look around you, see what's around, take a walk enjoy the surroundings, spend these next few minutes exploring your surroundings and feeling relaxed and happy. This is your time Paul, enjoy it. Now breathe very deeply and be aware of your breath. Feel the air rushing into your lungs and as you exhale I want you to sink deeper and deeper into the sofa, keep breathing in, then out, keep breathing and be conscious of every breath you take." I have to admit her voice engulfed you in some sort of sound blanket, it reassured you. For the first time in five months I was actually sitting on the sofa nice and relaxed, my breathing was natural but very deep; my mind was relaxed as all it saw was the sea. With my eyes shut I was able to transmit myself into the beautiful world that was Fistral Beach. I felt the sand and the sun, my shoulders relaxed and softened; my neck lost all its tension. I actually felt good. I lay there in this perfect state of relaxation, even the cats purred in unison, they were on the beach with me as well. With my eyes still closed, Martha got up and left the room. I was aware of this, but I really did not care. I was aware of her footsteps leaving the room, walking up the stairs and then I heard a door open and then close. Still in my perfect state of nirvana I then heard a noise that did not belong. As if someone had a huge jug of water and pouring it at a great height into the sink. There aren't any water falls on Fistral Beach. What the hell was it?

I opened my eyes and then realised that Martha was taking the longest piss I have ever heard just above me in her loo. My Fistral Beach disappeared quicker than you can say bog roll and I was very much back in the room with two cats on my lap and a CD player still churning out whale sounds. She stopped pissing, I heard the toilet roll being pulled, so good to see that she wipes and then the chain was pulled. She washed her hands and I heard her make her way down the stairs. I closed my eyes and sunk back in the sofa. I pretended that I had not noticed, and lay there in my fake trance. "Okay, I am going to count backwards from five and on each count I want you to breathe in and slowly come back to me in the room. Five . . ." As she slowly counted backwards I obliged with the breathing. All I could hear was her pissing away in my head. Fistral Beach was long gone I can tell you, and on one I opened my eyes. "How do you feel?"

"I feel fine", I responded, "I feel more relaxed." She smiled. I knew that was the reaction she wanted. She looked at her watch and said it was over and we should book another appointment.

I realised over the coming weeks that Martha actually spoke a lot of sense. What was really apparent were my anger issues with my company in that they had failed to do anything to help me. This was made worse when I got my first piece of contact from them. It was a letter from payroll telling me my pay was being decreased from over £500 per week down to statutory sick pay of only £72 per week. Also, just to add fuel to my fire, they were late sending me this notification and I owed them over £2000. But not to worry as I could pay this back in instalments. The reason for this was that they had continued paying me full pay after four months and it was now five months and I had not qualified for that yet. That's nice of them I thought. Well actually I did not think that at all. I rang my union representative and screamed and shouted like a crazy bald banshee down the phone at him and he assured me he would put this right. We had to wait for a meeting with the management, he would let me know when it was and all I had to do was sit and wait. Sitting and waiting for appointments became my full time job after this. I reckon I could have got a gold medal in the Olympics if they had the sitting and waiting category. No one rushed, no one seemed to care and every day I waited for an appointment to sort things I would fall into decline. I became very paranoid and really believed everyone was trying to screw me over. I mean, come on, here I was in a situation totally not my fault. All I was doing was my job, then explosion and then left out to dry. Not only did I see it that way at the time, as time went on I was proved to be more and more correct. It was hell.

However, I got the payroll letter the same day as an appointment with Martha. She let me in and I assumed the sofa position along with my moggy friends. She could see how agitated I was and naturally asked me what was wrong. I leant forward and said nothing, I just reached out and handed her the letter. As she looked at the letter her eyes opened, she stared straight back at me and said, "Oh."

"Oh? Is that all you got?" I angrily replied.

"Well what can I say? I cannot make this right. Have you spoken to them?" I told her how I was waiting for the meeting with some sort of management. She nodded her head, realising I needed some sort of reassurance.

"The thing is Paul, it's a huge organization. I am sure this is a computer printed letter that no one has even looked at, no one knows what happened to you in payroll; it's a completely different office.

Once they know I am sure it will be sorted." She was absolutely right: I had my meeting with management, they put things right and I got my money paid to me. The two things she taught me more than anything else is that firstly I am a number, or was a number. We all are really. No matter what happens in life, whether it be with doctors, solicitors, DHSS etc. etc. we are all just a file with a number. We have no face, no feelings and no one cares. They do their job with the least amount of minimum fuss and that's it; you are filed away and stored on a hard drive or a filing cabinet until the next time. The second thing she taught me was, "Shit happens," and boy was she right. The problem is, if someone tries to screw you over or indeed make your life miserable by not doing their job properly then what can you really do? We never saw eye to eye on this one , but over the last four years it has slowly sank in as I dealt with one idiot after another who thought they were the bees knees in their job.

Again at the end of the session as I lay there in my trance, whales calling out, waves crashing on the beach and some hippy type playing a Spanish guitar, off she would go up the stairs for her ritual piss. I wondered if she knew how thin her floors and walls were and why did she piss at the exact same time on each appointment? I reckon it was the waves and whales that set off. Each week as I was on my paradise beach in Cornwall off she would pop, up the stairs and let rip. It was so loud. I wondered if she had the most amazing powerful bladder squirting water out like a jet wash for cars or if she actually stood on the toilet seat to get maximum distance for noise affect. It ruined the affect each week but, I have to say, out of all my treatment she was by far the best. She never spoke down to me, she accepted what I said at face value, helped me deal with my negativity in a very strong way and challenged me with common sense. Some days we argued but nine times out of ten she won. She knew what she was talking about and handled everything perfectly. I would leave her feeling calmer and seeing things in a different light.

Like all good things they have to come to an end. My six sessions with Martha seemed to fly by. On the last day we had a good chat before I would hear her discharges from her bladder for the last time. "Paul, you have a severe anger management problem, clinical depression and post-traumatic stress, you have got to see a psychiatrist and get more ongoing help. I know someone who can help you, but he is private. Maybe your employers will pay?" I did not hold out much hope, but she agreed to write to my occupational health doctor with her recommendations and fingers crossed this would get the ball started for real help. I needed to move further down the conveyor belt and Martha was going to help me.

I must say I missed her words of wisdom, and on many occasion I wanted to go back to her again as so much crap was seeming to control my life and she helped me make sense of it all. I drove away for the last time, and it would nine months before I had any treatment again.

Chapter 6 - Therapy, therapy, where for art thou therapy?

It seemed like an eternity before any more treatment was arranged for me. This was the period of time that my home became more and more like a cage. The bars were of my own making; no matter what I tried to do I just could not go out and face walking into the street or even getting into my car. After every argument and screaming match I had down the telephone trying to get my treatment sorted, I would plummet down into a depressive episode that could last for days, even weeks. It was as if every ounce of energy I had would be put into trying to be heard by my company and, when got I nowhere, the frustration and anger of having no control over my life eventually made me realise I was completely helpless. I felt like I was banging my head against a brick wall. No matter how much I begged and asked for help no one was going to give me any answers. Then out of nowhere someone contacted me from my employers and agreed to arrange treatment, finally. What I should have done was to arrange NHS treatment off my own back and just waited in line like everyone else.

The problem was I was in a very weird situation; let me explain. As my company had basically admitted to screwing up my life they agreed to pay for my treatment and this meant I could bypass any waiting lists. They made out that nothing was too good for their drivers and they would do all they could to get me back in the driving seat and sort my life out. You name it and it would be there. It is a shame they didn't actually mean it. Like a fool I believed them, despite all the initial delays. So they contacted a private hospital about 20 miles away from me and arranged for me to see Dr Johnson, who apparently Martha had recommended I see. Now as it was private you would think book an appointment and just turn up and away we go. Oh no, my company wanted to know exactly how much it was all going to cost before they agreed to pay for it. Of course the hospital's response was, well we do not know what is wrong with him so we will have to see him and diagnose his problem. These sort of conversations were being done by letter, not email or phone but by bloody letter, so weeks and weeks would pass by while I still could not even get an initial appointment.

Despite my desperate calls to my union representative and to various managers, nothing would ever speed things up. "Oh it's up to accounts to say if they will pay for it." or "Oh I am not dealing with it anymore, it's all up at head office." So I ring head office, the response, "Oh that's being dealt with by your line manager locally, have you rung him?" So I ring him, "Oh that's with accounts now, we should hear any week now." and then it was, "Just waiting for someone to sign it off and you can go." Not only was I severely ill, suffering with extreme depression, post-traumatic stress with severe anxiety but they were adding anger management to my list. Everyone I called up on the telephone I would shout at. I would scream and scream and scream until finally they caved in and I actually got my appointment. Of course this meant over time fewer and fewer people would want to deal with me. I may have sounded unreasonable but this was my life they were playing with and when you are a number in a huge company, no one really cares. It actually took longer than waiting on the National Health Service. Then one day I get a letter in the post and an appointment is made.

So, off I went to the hospital. It was very daunting; I had never seen a psychiatrist before, I had not got a clue what was going to happen. The only thing I knew of shrinks was what was seen on TV; boy was I shitting myself. As I drove up to the car park I passed a beautiful pond with an amazing weeping willow leaning over the glass like water. There were ducks and their ducklings swimming in a row, it was a beautiful sight. I was early so I sat by the pond and waited until it was five minutes before my appointment and then in I went. This would be the first of what seemed like a million forms I had to fill in over the coming years. Every appointment you had to sign a disclaimer or write down your credit card details. I always left it blank and every time I said that my company was paying for it. The one thing these hospitals are quick off the mark at is getting your money, regardless if the treatment works or not.

I sat in the posh waiting room, with free cappuccino machines and spring water dispensers. On the table were magazines like Tattler, Country Life and horsy magazines. No sign of a 1978 Woman's Own and Tit Bits; these were even the same year and month. Definitely a place for posh mad people; not your typical working class type mad person like me.

Finally a slim gaunt figure appeared from a corridor and introduced himself to me. I followed him back to his room and sat down in front of desk. He had a huge oak wood desk with oak wood book cabinets all around, a lovely view of the grounds, a fountain pen and one of those leather blotting paper holders in front of him and more alarm presses you could shake a stick at. I just could not imagine any of these upper class mad people trying to lash out at him, I mean what would they use? A bottle of Chablis and a sharpened baguette? I mean, come on, maybe it's when they get the bill, "How much, you fucking bastard, one will smash ones face in you cad."

He went through all, what I soon learnt to be, standard type questions. He asked me about my parents, mental history, had I had depression before, did I take drugs, my alcohol intake, my home life and we just had about three minutes left to talk about the crash. He was very smart, because he realised that my depression had started soon after the crash and, this is the smart bit, because I did not have depression before the crash, it must have been the crash that had in some way affected me. Well hale fucking luya. Duh, do you think so? Who would have imagined?

So it was official. I am mad. I left with the diagnosis of post-traumatic stress, depression and anxiety disorder. He even prescribed me a wonderful drug that had the most amazing side effects. Death and anal leakage were on the list of side effects, so I was quite worried. The funny thing was the first treatment he recommended for me was a group therapy session for anger management. He said by the time I would start these sessions the drugs should have kicked in and this will attack my illness two pronged, using the amazing CBT techniques along with turning me into a sweaty miserable fucked up zombie in the process. Seemed ideal. The problem I had was that none of this could go ahead without my company agreeing to all the costs. So it was all added up and sent to them. This, needless to say, took more weeks. Then there were a few more weeks, as the appropriate people were on holiday and of course there was absolutely no one else in the whole wide world who could make any decision. I had to wait for this person, and I did not even know who this person was.

Two months went by, so I was back on the phone screaming and shouting to all the wrong people as no one would tell me who the right person was. The thing was they did not realise how much damage they were doing to me. I was in a bad place, and every call that said they couldn't help me was like a punch in the guts. It made me feel so worthless. This company who I was working for, earning money for them while getting badly injured, did not want anything to do with me whatsoever. They just didn't care. They had plenty of other drivers who could cover my work and get the overtime, so, me not being there was not a problem. So much for, nothing is too good for our drivers. So over a period of time I was forgotten, just left to rot in my new found cage, my house. My only support was my wife, who had had all this thrown on her lap as well. We did not know how to deal with it. Our moods went from bad to worse, she still had to go to work and I was left at home 10 hours a day all alone with so many negative thoughts running through my head. Without any treatment coming anytime soon I became very ill indeed. So bad I eventually called the private hospital and spoke to Dr Johnson's secretary to ask what was going on. All I wanted was an answer; all I wanted was some help. Then she explained to me what had been going on. The hospital had quoted a price for my treatment and they had said it was too much.

My employers even asked to try and reduce the amount of treatment I needed to bring the cost down. I mean that's like asking a nurse to bandage only half the broken leg so you don't have to pay for all the bandages, I mean, how fucking stupid is that? She then dropped a bombshell on me that sent me into an incredible rage: she said that they made it clear there was no way they were going to pay and that I should go back to my GP to seek NHS treatment. This had taken nearly five months. I had one assessment and that was it. Five months of being pushed from pillar to post, five months of complete uncertainty. It was hell, I just felt so low, I did not care what happened to me. My whole life was in turmoil and for once I was not the one who could make the changes. I needed help. I had never been like this before, it was a terrifying time and every argument on the phone caused a rage in me that I had never felt before. I wanted the person dead, anyone who dared cross my path would get so much abuse it would be intolerable for the person concerned and they would hang up. I would cause arguments in order to make them respond; it was the only way. I did not want anyone to treat me like shit, but I was too low and weak to react properly and deal with things normally. All I knew was to lash out. I wanted to hurt them like they were hurting and destroying me. The problem was I was just a folder on a desk to them, when they put the phone down it was forgotten or passed to the next person. In that folder was my life, my financial security, my state of mind and my health and they did not care.

The drugs I was on were supposed to stop that. The wonderful side affects sure made me a catch for the ladies I can tell you. Not only did I sweat like a pig's arse morning, noon and night it also made my paralysis on the side of my mouth drool. Very attractive don't you think? The only good thing about this was I was suffering from such bad anxiety I barely went out of the house. I rang Dr Johnson's secretary and asked him if I could change them, but he replied, "I cannot interfere now as you are under NHS treatment so you will have to wait till you see someone there." Great. I just stopped taking them. I didn't care. If you medication, please do not do this as it really does do more damage. Make sure you stop the medication in a controlled way. All that happened to me was that my mood plummeted, I became irrational and, for some reason, my muscles felt like they had turned to concrete. I would not mind if I looked buff but I didn't: the steroids I was taking to improve the nerves in my head were really making me pile on the weight. I was much fatter, more depressed than ever and slowly becoming more and more isolated from the rest of my world.

Things just could not get any worse, and then there was a letter posted through my front door. It was from my company. It was proof to me that there was a devil and there was a hell and my personnel and payroll people from my company lived there. It read:

Dear Mr. Holmes,

As you are aware you have been on sick leave for a period of six months while still receiving full pay. Under the last pay agreement, you would normally now receive half pay for the next six months. However, as you have not been with this company for five years you were only entitled to four months' full pay and your wages will now go down to statutory sick pay of £72.00 per week. This means we have also in error paid you two months' wages too much meaning you will have to pay back £2700. Please can you contact us to arrange payment?

You could not make it up could you? I now owed my company over £2000 because I was in a crash at work that was their fault. Not only was my main income stopping but I was now in debt. I held the letter in my hand staring at the words, re-reading it over and over again, making sure it was not my depression distorting the words. Then from a complete numbness and state of shock I exploded into a rage never seen by anyone before. I grabbed my phone and rang the payroll number. Amazingly I was able to give them my details before throwing abuse after abuse at them down the phone "What the fuck do you think you are doing?" and more words to that effect. As usual they were not the people to speak to. I would have to speak to my line manager, my line manager said he could not authorize me getting full pay and it would have to go to a director of some sort. All this took more and more time and of course took its toll on me.

I was being placed in the situation where I could only earn my wages if I was well enough to work. If you can't work then you are damaged goods and no good to anyone. How on earth can I get back to work when all they were doing was withholding my treatment? It was a vicious circle; the more they neglected my treatment the worse I became which meant I became less likely to go back to work. I did not trust them, I hated them with a passion. I do not even have the words to explain. How could they do this to me? The fact was I could not even live a normal life: I could not sleep, eat, drink, concentrate or function in any shape or form without the help of some drug. How the hell was I going to go back to the railway and slot back to work? I had had no treatment because of them, they had delayed it, and now I was paying for it. I hated the bastards. I wanted them dead. How dare they treat me like a worthless piece of human scrap? I was a payroll number and nothing else, I realised this. Slowly I began to realise in the big scheme of things I was completely worthless and I felt every bit of it, every single bit.

In the end I rang my union representative and he arranged a meeting with a manager who had obviously been given instructions on what to say. We all sat down and came to an agreement that I would return to full pay but it would be reviewed each month. That meant each month's pay could be my last but I would not know until it did not come through to my bank. How did they expect me to live like that? I could not plan past 28 days: the railway pay four-weekly. I needed to have the security behind me but that had been taken away from me, now I just did not have a clue what the hell was going to go on. I was worried about my health, my state of mind and now my mortgage, loans and the security for my wife and I. All they were doing was adding insult to injury and they did not care one jot.

Soon after this I got an appointment with an NHS psychiatrist. Thankfully it was a morning appointment so I did not have to dwell on it all day. I had for some reason got into a habit where I could only do one thing on a day. So if I had an appointment on a certain day I could not arrange or do anything else. It was as if all my energies would be spent on that one action. So if the appointment was at the end of the day, I would be a complete anxious wreck all day not eating, drinking and just sitting there waiting for the time to come round when I had to go. When I would come out of the appointment it was like a release, I could relax and return to what was my normality.

As described in chapter three, I had to meet a very young Asian senior house officer; not the real psychiatrist, obviously I was not worthy of such treatment, I mean you had to be completely bonkers to see one of them after all. She was a very timid young lady who, and mean this with no disrespect, was not right for this sort of work. Not because English was not her first language or because she was Asian or a woman, she was just so wrong. All she would do is read out questions off a clipboard and write the answers down. When she got down to the bottom of the page she would go out of the room and return five minutes later with a fresh batch of questions. Each time she left the room she would leave her handbag on her desk. It was wide open with her purse and hospital ID on full display; she obviously did not have a clue.

After she allowed me to have depression with post-traumatic stress I made it quite clear I was not happy just seeing her and I wanted to see a psychiatrist. I mean, after all that's why I was there. I was asked to go and sit back in the waiting room and when she had time I would be called in. We all know that any NHS waiting room is the pits. Bolted down chairs, bullet proof glass for the receptionists who all behave like little Hitler's. You are never ever seen on time even if you are the first appointment

A MAN DERAILED

of the day. Why is that? I always book the first appointment of the day and I am always kept waiting for 20 minutes or so; if it was the last appointment you could understand. I mean twenty minutes is a long time in a National Health Service mental clinic. Believe me, it can be quite scary. This is another trait of depression: you have high expectations on everyone else and no one ever seems to match them. It sort of turns you into a snob of sorts, it's not good. So I sat back in the waiting surrounded by all the weird and wonderful patients of my local area, they looked dishevelled, they looked unclean and they looked very ill. The sad thing was I fitted in just fine. I sat there in my jogging bottoms, tee shirt and trainers with no socks. We all know what happens to trainers after a few weeks of wearing them with no socks don't we? Oh yes, we burn them. I was unshaven , I felt as if the beard would cover my paralysed face, but to be honest I just looked like I had a lop sided beard and if anything it highlighted it more.

At last I was called in to see Dr Wooley. She was a hippy sort and was not very happy about me undermining her staff and demanding to see a real psychiatrist. She sat behind her desk with her arms folded and asked me how she could help.

"I just do not feel putting me on antidepressants for three months and coming back to see how I am is good enough. I was supposed to have cognitive behavioural therapy with Dr Johnson. I mean, can we not do that here?" She looked at me as if I had asked for the crown jewels to be placed on my lap.

"Well," she replied, "I can put you on the list if you want, but I haven't got a clue when it would start for you, it could be six months."

"It would be nine months if I waited to come back in three months and asked then wouldn't it?" I replied. She agreed to put me on the list and sent me away with my lovely little prescription slip.

So you see one minute I was a private patient and then I was thrown back to the mercy of the NHS. The NHS may be slow but at least I was in their system and that meant things will slowly start to turn around.

Just to add another thread to this tale, I had to see my occupational health doctor as well. She was paid by my employers to assess me every six weeks. Dr Kenny was a very pale lady who spoke with such a soft voice I would sometimes not even realise she was talking. She actually showed great concern for me but could only make recommendations. Basically she would write a report saying this man needs help, send it to my employers and they would file it away. I hated seeing her for two reasons; firstly I always knew it was a waste of time, as my employers never did what she said they should do. Basically she said I needed loads of treatment and the only way to get me back behind the controls of a train anytime soon was to get it done privately. Secondly, it was a two hour journey to visit her. I had to travel all the way up to north west London. They made me go on the trains that I was anxious about, the trains I feared, and then I had to get on a tube just to get there. By the time I arrived I was always a complete wreck. On one particular appointment with her, she was adamant that she was not going to let them hold back my treatment anymore. She was going to write a serious letter and make sure it started as soon as possible. I nodded as she spoke. These sessions that I had to travel for two hours each way only lasted less than five minutes so I went in, nodded my head and went home. I thought it would be yet another waste of time.

Then a pig flew past my window. Well it might as well have done. I suddenly got a letter from the private hospital saying I had been discharged from the care, laughable care, of Dr Wooley and was back in the care of Dr Johnson. I had been assigned a psychotherapist, her name was Penny, and she was going to see me for one to one sessions and also run my group therapy for anger management. It was all going to start the following week. I could not believe it, Dr Kenny had done something, and I was extremely grateful. My treatment was going to start at long last. Another three months and it would have been two years since the crash. Oh how time flies when you are having such fun.

One question I get asked a lot is, what is the difference between a psychiatrist and a psychotherapist? Now that's easy. It's about £50 per hour. Sorry, I could not resist. A therapist is more hands on so to speak. Basically they will go through all the problems one by one and talk you though them. They may even be a bit human by saying things like "Oh no, that's awful," or "Well you did well to deal with that." They may use a tool called cognitive behavioural therapy. This is a way of challenging your negative thoughts; more on that later. A psychiatrist is more blunt and more matter of fact. They will ask you set questions, work a diagnosis which can never be wrong in a million years and then pass you over to your therapist. Once the treatment's over you will be assessed again and the process goes on. One of the things that the psychiatrist can do is to prescribe medication. I was still on the medication that Dr Wooley prescribed and its biggest side affect was that I never felt full after meals no matter how much I ate or drank. Not good when you are still taking steroids. I did not sweat as much as the ones before or indeed slur, but I had turned into Pac man, wanting to eat everything that moves. Needless to say the weight piled on. In conjunction with these I was on a mild sleeping tablet that added an extra hour or two onto my sleep pattern and, I have to be honest, I was quite happy with that. I was sick of those 3 am starts and sitting there for three or four hours waiting for the rest of the world to catch up with me.

So, after months and months of wrangling, here I am walking past the most beautiful pond and weeping willow. Again the ducks were there, but I was probably looking at the ducklings from the year or so before who had all grown up and were no doubt laying their own eggs. Again I sat next to the cappuccino machine and saw it had a hot chocolate button. I thought what the hell, let's throw caution to the wind. It was a huge step for me as I never drank in public if I could help it. I hate the dribbling from my paralysed side of my mouth. However, I was the only one here and I felt daring. The brown liquid squirted into the cup and as soon as it stopped I pulled out a frothy hot chocolate. No sooner had I sat down again, Penny appeared and introduced herself and off we went to her room. She was as easy to talk to as Martha was and did not keep disappearing off for a wee at the end of the session so that was a bonus. She then explained to me about my anger management group therapy that she was running, she told me about the group exercises we would be doing and also that if I had any worries whatsoever to talk to her and she would kindly address them for me.

So for the next four weeks we would solely be concentrating on my anger management techniques using CBT (cognitive behavioural therapy). I had heard great things about CBT so I was very pleased to finally get the chance to learn about it and put it into use. To simplify it, basically you discuss a scenario that is making you angry (of course it could be depressed or anxious), you then talk it through and work out how angry you are. You say on a scale of 100 you are 95. You talk the situation through and realise it's not that bad and you say ok, on a scale of 100 I am now about 40. Job done. Apparently for many this works and in Penny's room it did work. I could happily tell her what was making me angry, mainly my employers. We listed them, applied these techniques and off I went all happy knowing my anger levels were nice and low. The problem I found with CBT was that I could not use it at the actual time the things were making me angry, well because I was so bloody angry. I would see red, scream and shout like a complete and utter mad thing, make sure my point was made and then leave the situation wanting to blow everyone's head off with a sodding shotgun. When I had calmed down naturally I would use CBT and realised that decapitating my management and putting their heads up on spikes and then marching around the town to show the other people what happens to you when you try to shit on me, was a little over the top. I would work my way down to just shooting them, then punching them, then having a damn good conversation to thrash out the problem to I really do not give shit anymore. CBT did not control the feelings I had at the time in my chest and did not stop my outbursts. It did make me think and over time I could see the obstacles I had to overcome to try and avoid these situations. So really what I was taught was avoidance. This meant not opening mail, answering the door, or indeed calling anyone or answering the phone. Let's be honest, you cannot live like that. The only way I was going to be calm and ok was if I got treated properly by my management and that wasn't going to happen.

So the day of the group sessions came and I was extremely nervous. This meant opening up in front of complete strangers and, I have to be honest, I did not sleep for two nights before the start. When I got to the hospital I was a wreck, I was unshaven, had sunken eyes and looked like crap. I was in the best place so that was handy. I sat in the waiting room and waited for my other fellow angry acquaintances to appear. I resisted the hot chocolate as I was feeling sick. I soon became even more anxious as I was still the only one in the waiting room and it was supposed to start in the next few minutes. I went out to reception to check I was in the right place. I deliberately got there early to make sure I did not walk into a room last and everyone turn round and look at me; that was a nightmare for me. I hated being centre of attention. I still do. I just cannot deal with it. I become so anxious I can hardly speak and therefore feel stupid and want the whole earth to open and swallow me up. It was ok, I was in the right place, and then in walked Penny looking somewhat embarrassed and sheepish. She looked at me and smiled, "Shall we go over to the room, Paul?" I followed her, my anxiety was going through the roof, the sweats, why didn't I get here earlier, I must have been in the wrong place the bloody receptionist was wrong, damn damn damn.

I cannot walk into a room full of people, I can't, I got to go. I wanted to run as far away as I could. She went to a door, she pushed it open. My anxiety rate was 99 for those of you who understand CBT. As she opened the door I could see there was no light on. She turned it on and all there was in there was a desk and a couple of chairs. "Take a seat, Paul." She opened a window and put her files on the desk. She then looked at me and said, "I am afraid you are the only one who has turned up; it's just going to be you and me." Apparently all of them had either rung in sick or changed their minds so, from eight of us, it was just me. My CBT anxiety level was 28 at this point.

Over the following weeks I had learned how to take steps in curbing my outbursts. Basically you are taught shit happens, deal with it. I know that sounds somewhat cynical and it is. I am a very cynical person. I had to be. I guess it's a safeguard to stop others from hurting you or trying to shit on you. The big question was, are my employers being unreasonable or am I over-acting? Is the anger and rage I was experiencing justifiable? Well yes actually. My problem was not so much how I was being treated at this point in time, it was all the bullshit they fed me by telling me no matter what I need to get my back on my feet , they were there. Like hell, if it was free then fine, but if it meant paying for anything then you are on your own. "Wait." I hear you shout, "Aren't they paying for your anger management treatment?" Yes they were, and jolly nice it was too. Lots of frothy coffee and filling in CBT forms, and some homework now and then as well. All good stuff and helpful. There was a week in-between each session.

Each week I would turn for my solo group therapy and Penny would ask me, "So, Paul, how was your week?" Three hours later I would stop moaning about what had happened during that week. I felt sorry for Penny, it must have bored her to tears. Every now and then, as I stopped for a breath, she would try to interject a positive little note like, "Well I am sure they didn't mean to do that" and I would reply, "Of course they did, why else would they do it?" My argument to all my anger was simple. They had a choice whether to piss me off or not, they had a choice whether they should send down into a depressed state, to make me anxious. It was a conscious decision by another human being. There were things like not coming back to me with answers I needed, or not having arranged a report that needed doing, or sorting out my wages. One thing after another I seemed to be chasing to get done, and I was getter more and more angry. My employers just did not have a clue and as for my union, they did not have clue. Out of sight out of mind, that's how large companies work, until your file pops up on someone else's desk and they say, "Hey, what's happening with this Holmes bloke?"

My anger management therapy had finished. The four weeks flew by and, though I felt more or less the same, I seemed to be able to bottle it up long enough for me not to snap back and walk away. All it seemed to do was to make me more agreeable to everyone else no matter how I felt. The drugs are the same as well. You are given them to make your behaviour more acceptable to others. I do not agree with that as it masks the real problems lurking beneath. How many people live like zombies just because it suits the neighbours or the family? Don't get me wrong, we have to protect others but do it properly. Do not take away the quality of life that we all deserve just so we cannot be an irritant for someone else, it's so wrong.

Anyway, off I went and waited for my next course of therapy. It was going to be a depression group therapy class so, as you can imagine, it would be a right laugh. They had told me there would be a gap of a couple of weeks so off I went practicing my new found cognitive behavioural therapy techniques. They must have worked as during the next two weeks it was quite uneventful, hence why I have skipped through to the depression therapy. I mean I didn't kill anyone in the Co-op, I didn't want to smother the mail man who has a habit of delivering parcels at my house at 6 am stinking of roll up cigarettes. I deliberately did not contact my employers for anything; another month's money went into my account so I was secure for at least four weeks. So things were looking up.

I was not the first one in the waiting room this time: there were four men and four ladies. There was no huge ash tray in the middle of the room to throw your car keys in or any fondue sets, so just a normal waiting room and we were all depressed. As each one walked into the waiting room we all acknowledged each other, but barely making eye contact and that weird half smile as if to say "Ahhhh, you're nuts too?" It was only a half smile for me too as half my mouth still was not working properly. So in we go and are confronted with a semicircle of chairs and the usual flip chart up against the wall. I sat in the middle chair. One thing I had always learnt on any course no matter what you were trying to learn whether it be corporate, night school or any training thing, if you sat at the end you would always be picked on to answer questions first at some point in the proceedings. Now, in the middle you would always have more time before they get to you to answer no matter which end they start. Smart huh? We are given name tags and are asked to stick them to our clothes, top half of course, so we all know who each other is. On the end of the semicircle is a very unkempt man called Ken. He really looked like he was about to shoot himself. The act of writing those three letters on the stickers seemed to have taken it all out of him and he sat there with his head in his hands, mumbling under his breath. He was not happy and let's face it, he was in the right place. So let's get ready to rumble. It's time to destroy my depression, I am in the right chair, got my badge with my name on, I am a fruit loop the scene was set.

Jane, our therapist for the day, stood up in front of us and said, "Good morning everyone, I am Jane and I am going to be your therapist for the day. I shall be guiding you through our techniques we use for allowing you to tackle your depression. It's called Cognitive Behavioural Therapy. Firstly, I want us all to share a little as to why we are here. So Paul, why you don't you start?" Shit, I could not believe it, not only was I going to have to be the first one to talk but I also had to go through all this CBT yet again. I was like a deer in headlights but I managed to say my little monologue and then, when I had finished, the relief was huge. My face filled with blood with embarrassment, and slowly it returned to normal as everyone else started to tell their stories. I could not really believe how much confidence I had lost. I used to be able to talk in front of people but, having spent so much time in solitary in my house I slowly grew to call my cage, I realised how much it had taken its toll on me.

"OK, thank you. Now, Ken, how about you?"

"No." he abruptly replied.

"Why Ken, what's wrong?"

"Who cares? Does anyone here really care? I am better off dead." The group went completely silent; I mean, what do you say to that? "Yes Ken, you are." No, of course not. None of us could take our eyes off him as he buried his face into his hands.

"How about we have a 15 minute break? Everyone back here at 10.30 please." We all got up and walked back to the waiting rooms for the coffee machine and then, one by one, we went out into the garden where the pond was. Immediately everyone except me pulled out a cigarette and smoked it as quick as they could so they could get a second one in their mouth before we had to go back in.

We all went back to the treatment room. This time there was only seven. Ken had gone. "Right, let's start shall we?" Jane said as she walked in through the door. One of the others quickly pointed out that Ken was not here and shouldn't we wait?

"Ken will not be joining us I am afraid, he would bring the whole group down and this is not what we are about today. So everyone grab a pen and . . ."

A MAN DERAILED

Ken had been kicked off a depression therapy session for being too depressed. I remember thinking that was harsh but he would have made the sessions seem like hell there are no two ways about it. I do hope they arranged something else for him, I never did find out.

So off I go on the CBT course work yet again. Again, it just did not work for me, the things that were making me depressed were external problems and still continuing from my employers and various other bits and bobs. What was needed was for everything else to change and I would be ok. However, I was informed that was not going to happen so I would have to learn how to deal with it. I soon learnt the planet earth would be so much better without humans, oh well, not going to happen. So another four weeks came and went. I had found it very hard to talk in group therapy. I had spent so much time home alone that I had really lost my skills of talking to other people, especially in front of other people. If I had to give out an answer I was aware of the other people looking at me. It made me stutter, it made me feel stupid and I really hated it. I dreaded each session and I was relieved when it had finished. I had to be honest, I got sick and tired of hearing everyone else's problems. I know that sounds really selfish, but depression does that, it does make you very inward looking and at this point of time in my life I felt like I was fighting to keep my career, my marriage and every other significant piece of my life. Hearing the other people's problems just did not do it for me especially as one of the men, Chris, in his late fifties, kept saying the whole time, "I really do not know why I am here, I feel great." So he would not open up when talking. It later transpired that he had a heart attack, a bad one by all accounts. Can you have good ones? He spent ages in hospital and lost a career and was put out on pastures new. Basically they retired him early. At first he found the adjustment extremely hard to cope with but now he'd got a boat and spent his days sailing and basically having a lovely time on one of the east Essex's rivers. It all sounded quite idyllic to me. However, I don't think he realised how much the trauma of having the heart attack affected him and he was trying to keep this good old stiff upper lip thing. "Well if it happens again I will know what to expect, I have had a good innings," all that sort of nonsense to be honest, but to be frank I think he was petrified it was going to happen again. He was just too scared to admit it. I hope he is still sailing, he was a nice chap.

So, as you can imagine, I knew CBT like the back of my hand what with eight weeks of using it, filling out forms and telling others how it prevented me from losing my temper or how it made me get up and do stuff without letting depression hold me back. The real reason I felt better was nothing to do with the CBT and that was not the CBT's fault, it was that I had been meeting other people and integrating with them. I had suddenly felt like I was not alone and that I was not the only one who was suffering all this crap and torment. It did not matter why it had happened and when, all that mattered was I knew I was not the only struggling with depression. The condition makes you feel that way, it makes you feel lonely and distant, and it makes you feel like you are the only person in the world not laughing or smiling at this particular time. Here were six others that proved that wrong and when we had lunch in the hospital canteen there were another 40 there that proved it; these poor souls were even worse than me. At least I could survive in the real world but these people could not. They walked around in their dressing gowns, looking like they were scared out of their wits and that was no hope for them. This was a private hospital for God's sakes, beautiful gardens, a gym, their own TVs in their own rooms, family coming whenever they want to but what were they like in NHS ones, I could not bear to think. So I learnt a lesson, I was not alone. It did not make me feel good, it just made me realise that maybe the grass is not always greener.

So on to anxiety, and anxiety is not a pleasant thing to experience. The hospital had penned me in for some more treatment but I had to have a one to one session with my psychiatrist to see where we were at. Again Dr Johnson met me in the waiting room and again we sat down surrounded by oak furniture and twee wallpaper. He then made a rather brilliant suggestion: he said I should go back to work in some sort of capacity while having some sort of treatment running parallel so I could keep on getting the support. So the anxiety treatment was placed on hold and my work was contacted about me going back to some sort of administration role. As usual my employers dragged their feet but eventually they came up with a job that I should be able to handle. Basically I had to go to four locations and collect time sheets and replace them with new ones for the drivers to sign in when they start work. Well that seemed easy enough. So I happily agreed. The good thing was this also meant my salary would then automatically continue to get paid and I could slowly integrate back into the work place. Along with this I would have weekly sessions with my therapist to keep me as sane as possible.

So the morning came when I had to go and sign on and perform my first day's work in what seemed like a lifetime. It was one of those damp November mornings, all misty and loads of moisture in the air. I drove to my depot and parked up. I had severe anxiety, purely because I knew the signing on depot would be full of drivers. They would all want to know how I was and no doubt ask me loads of questions. The problem with the railway is that it does suffer with Chinese whispers. So someone would tell another driver that I was involved in an accident with the overhead power lines and was injured, then after it had been recycled by 20 other drivers I was in a massive train wreck and lost both my legs and had severe burns. I parked up in the car park; it was so strange getting out of the car in my uniform and high visibility vest on. You had to wear the vest as you had to cross about 10 railway lines to get to the signing on point. In the dark and wet it is a very eerie place. The overhead power lines buzzed like mad as the moisture surrounded them. All the trains that were stabled there had their compressors churning over and over. The creaking of the air through the valves brought me back to the dark horrible night of my crash. I felt all the hairs on my neck stand up as if I had static electricity surrounding me. Sparks flew from the pantograph of a train as it moved out of the depot to begin its day's work. They were the same sparks that exploded in my face. All the sights and sounds of my crash lay before me. Then the smell of my burnt hair and skin came back to me, it was so vivid. I leaned forward and vomited, I was standing right on a train line at the time, I moved to a bush that was nearby and made the most awful retching noise. I had not eaten so all I was spitting up was bile. It burnt my throat and tasted awful. I ran the best I could over the tracks and into the depot. Thankfully the first room you come to is the gents' toilet so I barged in and locked myself in a stall. I had been transported back in time to that night; I felt the loneliness and helpfulness that made me feel so weak that night.

My chest was pounding, my uniform was saturated with sweat, I could not catch my breath, each time I breathed in I could taste my own bile, I kept gagging on the taste. I spat it all out in the toilet and checked there was no one else in the toilet. I rinsed my mouth out and splashed my face with water. This was a complete shock. I did not realise the whole environment would affect me like that. I spent ten minutes in the toilet trying to compose myself and then left to sign on. When I walked in many didn't know who I was, it had been that long since I had signed on for duty before. The few that did recognise me were very supportive and came up to me and asked me questions. They made me feel quite good. It was nice that they were keen to see I was ok and it was genuine; I was extremely grateful. I signed on and was a given a bundle of papers to distribute. I then left and had to negotiate walking back the way I came. I put my head down and walked as fast as I could. I almost ran up the platform and got on the next train that was going to pull out and off I went. Most people thought that because I could travel in a train ok that my bad reaction could not happen. I have to be honest, so did I. The thing is, in a train you are concealed, you cannot see the overhead power cables. You just see the platforms and all else around you. Ironically I felt safer in the passenger area of the train. It was just seats and a door at each end of the carriage; nobody took any notice of me.

I sat down and had about twenty minutes before my first stop. My anxiety receded and the rocking of the train helped me relax a bit. Before I knew it I had to get off and do my bit of administration and then wait for the next train. I had to do this four times. All in all it would take about four hours, ten minutes of which was the work and the rest of the time was the travelling to the various points. It was not hard, well it would not be if it was not for that first bit in the morning. I was determined to beat it. The next morning I did not need to wake up as I had been awake all night dreading this moment. Again I drove to the same car park, in the same parking space. Got out and the fear would grip me. I would try to walk fast, looking at my feet, jumping over train tracks and ballast, trying not to fall over but the fear would get me in the end. Each morning I had to vomit either before leaving for work or once I got there. My chest would feel like my heart was trying to jump out of my chest and my lungs just froze or were they breathing in and out so fast I didn't notice? It was extremely hard to tell. After my time composing myself I would walk in, sign on, and off I go again. I then had to go to my therapist to see how things were going on. Penny greeted me and sat me down. She smiled and asked me a very hopeful voice, "Well then, how's it been going?" I almost did not have the heart to tell her. I almost felt that if I said I was having vomiting fits every morning I would be saying the treatment was not working. I knew I could not go on like that so I told her. Her smile dropped to a frown and I felt as if I had failed. I had had thousands of pounds worth of treatment and here I am in a situation where I cannot even sign on at work without throwing up. It was not a good scenario. I told her I wanted to stick with it, maybe it would ease after a while, I really did not know but I knew I did not want to fail. The job was the easiest job in the world; surely I could not fail at this as well?

"I think you need to come on the anxiety class before going back to work. I will talk to Dr Johnson and see if he can arrange that for you. The class starts Monday so why not come on that and see how we go?" I knew that meant I would have to go sick again and once again I would be put in the situation of not knowing if I would get paid from one month to the next; I hated living like that. So I left the session with Penny and went home. I rang my supervisor and explained the situation and waited for Monday to come along.

Monday quickly came. I drove back up to the hospital and once again I sat in a waiting room with seven other strangers all nodding at each other and giving those embarrassing smiles as we waited to be called in. Then the receptionist came in and called my name out and asked me to go to the main desk.

She looked at me and said, "There seems to be a problem with funding for your treatment."

"Oh no it's ok, my company are paying for it. Dr Johnson has arranged it all." She shook her head as I spoke and handed me piece of paper. It was an email from my manager saying they were not prepared to pay for anymore treatment as this was not included in the original estimate.

"Do you have a credit card?" She asked.

"For how much?"

"Well's it's £800 for today and then each day thereafter."

"How much?" I shrieked, "you got to be kidding?" All this happening within earshot of the rest of the patients, how embarrassing.

Within ten minutes I was back in my car driving home. They had pulled my funding. I knew what was to follow, more arguments on the phone, again me never getting through to the right person, he is on holiday or not available. Guess what? That's exactly what I got. So I was left in limbo, no treatment, no job, not a clue of what was going to happen.

Three weeks had passed and boy was I in a complete state by this point. Then a letter plopped through my letter box and it was an appointment for me to meet a manager to discuss where we go from here. I rang my union representative and he said he would come with me. It was only a week away, so yet another week of anxiety and not knowing what the hell was going to happen. Waiting was the hard thing, days dragged and I was almost paralysed, unable to do anything in between all these appointments. For hours and hours, in my lonely depressed state, I would play out all the worst case scenarios in my head. It would affect the little sleep I had, making me have dreams where I would be forced to drive a train completely full with passengers and then it would fall off the same bridge in the high street. As usual I would wake at the same point in the dream and it would be 2 am. I could never get back to sleep. It drove me nuts.

I turned up at the meeting, there was a man from human resources, the manager and my union rep and I. Well I just sat there as they basically said there is no job for me and I cannot work within the railway environment so they were letting me go. Two days before Christmas and I was sacked. No fault of my own, just dropped like a piece of crap. I got ten weeks' money and a £1000 severance pay.

There would be no more treatment, no job, no wages, no more security. I had lost my identity. I was no longer an injured train driver, I was unemployed, depressed with no hope whatsoever.

I left the meeting; I was completely numb. How the hell was I going to explain it to my wife? I got home, sat down and cried. I cried for what seemed an eternity. A career I was hoping to keep for another 25 years had gone. I spent a whole year training for it, I even moved to the area for the job. My whole life revolved around this job before the crash. Now it had been taken away from me through no fault of my own. My state of mind plummeted, what the hell was I going to do?

A MAN DERAILED

Chapter 7 - Ahhh Solicitors . . . Don't you just love them?

This chapter is probably the weirdest, no hardest, episode to explain. Even as I sit here thinking how to explain it I still cannot believe it happened. However I shall try my best. I shall also keep the swearing down to a bare minimum, I promise, I will really try. I promise you, I did not make this up. I mean you could not make this up for God's sakes.

Well, with any injury these days someone has to pay for it. Well, eventually the insurers do but they do not meet you and say, "Oh you poor thing. Here, have some money and I hope this helps heal the pain." No, you need a solicitor then your employers need a solicitor and that's when things grind down to such a slow pace you begin to wonder if anything is actually happening at all. Generally it isn't, except for the law firms who are shovelling their money into suitcases and having a wonderful lifestyle out of all our misery. Gawd bless em.

My union instructed a firm of solicitors to act on my behalf. It was the one and only reason why I joined the union. The legal stuff you get with being member is generally quite good and now was the time when I needed their help. I was not sure what we were actually going to achieve at this point. As far as I was concerned I was going to have treatment, as my management promised me nothing was too good for their drivers, and then I would be back. So basically I would maybe get money for the injury caused to my face and the mental health issues. So I filled out my forms and sent them off to the solicitors and three months later I heard back from them. I got a letter arranging an appointment with a Henrietta Longsworth, oooooooo very posh I hear you cry, and so the time came to meet. She was nothing you would imagine her name would conjure up. Don't get me wrong, I have learnt ages ago not to go by appearances but she certainly should not have been called Henrietta, more like Deidre, sorry Deidre if you are reading this, nothing personal. She was clumsy as hell, carrying a huge folder with my name splashed all over it, papers flying all over the office as she dropped them. So much for data protection. It was a thick folder as well. How could it be so thick, I had only just got there? She pulled out a pad and pen and then asked me what happened. So I explained what had happened and at this point I was still waiting for treatment. She wrote it all down and then said, "Do you have home insurance?"

"Yes" I replied.

"Ok, well just in case we do not win the court case, we can claim our fees off your home insurance, so can you fill this in?" I was reluctant to do so and said I could not remember the details and I would forward them on. I never did. So that was it really, months went by and nothing happened. Every now and then I would get a letter with a form for me to fill in allowing them access to my GP notes and other medical history and that was it.

A MAN DERAILED

Then a really weird thing happened. I got a call from someone who will remain anonymous and they told me that the company who look after the whole infrastructure of the railway were having an inquiry about my accident but it was a closed one, meaning private, and I would not be attending and to top it all off it was the very next day. How the hell can they have an inquiry without me being there? It was typical of the railway though. They would cover up anything if they could. I got on to my management and asked what the hell was going on?

"How did you know?" was his reply.

"It doesn't matter how I know, what the hell is going on?" He agreed that he would be putting up a good fight for me, not that it was hard as I did not do anything wrong and he said he would share the findings with me when the report comes back. I really had little choice but to agree. No one wanted me there and to be honest I was not well enough to go up to London and face the people who had seemingly ruined my life.

A week later I got a call and my manager agreed to meet me and show me the findings of the inquiry. He had a draft report that had come back to him and he was quite happy for me to read it. So the next day I met him at some offices. It was quite hard for me to do, I had so much hatred for the managers not for anything that they had done personally but for all the stuff they had not done, like call me, see how I was and make sure I didn't need any help, but I soon learnt then when you are just known by your payroll number that sort of treatment is not going to happen. The quicker I accepted that the easier things would have been for me. The problem was I never did, and the more ill I got the more irrational and fierce my anger became towards them.

I sat in the office and my manager showed me the report. It was quite thick and it seemed like an age before I managed to get through it. It was mainly minutes from the meeting and, I have to admit, my manager spoke well for me and I was pleasantly surprised. The findings were all in my favour: I was travelling under 20 mph as per the rule book. I was given the wrong instructions by the signaller and after the explosion I did a reasonable job of disembarking the passengers and getting them to safety. I had to be honest I have not got a clue what happened during this time. It was weird reading a statement from the guard who was with me that night. After the explosion it was really him that did everything regarding the passengers. I was just in shock and working on autopilot. My memories are really of the explosion and then the time after everyone had gone and I was sitting there in the dark waiting for someone to come. There was one criticism of me that really got my back up and that was that I did not lay detonators behind my train. I shall explain. When you become a train driver, your whole life is to evolve around the book of rules and regulations. Before you can drive a train you spend six months learning this book inside and out before you can even get in the driving cab. Most of the rules were for bygone years when we had steam and semaphore signals (they are the signals that are like planks of wood moving up and down instead of the good old red yellow and green lights we have today). I am sure there is even a rule about where to put your shovel once you have filled up the furnace. I know what I would like to do with the shovel but that's another story and never happened, honest. So you learn the pages of this the most tedious book in the world, you learn hand signals, bell codes, what to do if this happens etc. etc. One of the things you have to do if you have had a situation is to protect your train. So basically you have to walk back a mile with these mini explosives, you then strap them to the railway track, so if any train behind you is hurtling towards you they will hear 3 explosions, this will frighten the shit out of the poor driver and he will automatically apply the brakes. I however did not do this and was criticised for it. I was not happy but rule are rules and it was not needed as all the trains on the running line could not be moved anyway as there was no power; it had all just earthed through my bloody cab.

So I had handed the report back to my manager and he asked what I had thought of it. I told him I was happy with what was said, especially the conclusion where it said I was not at fault one bit. I really thought they were going to put the blame on me, I mean why else would they not allow me to go and hear what was going on, but thankfully my fears were unfounded. So naturally I asked for a copy of the report, well you would wouldn't you? I mean here it is in black and white, saying it was everyone else's fault but mine. Why wouldn't I want a copy?

"I cannot do that, I was not even supposed to show you," he said,

"What do you mean you wasn't even supposed to show me? The bloody thing is about me."

"Look, we have these meetings to see if anything had gone wrong with the systems and make sure we learn from them. This is not for the outside, it stays here. I am sorry." I lost the plot to be honest with you. I smashed my fist down on the table and demanded he give me a copy, I was not going to leave until they gave me a copy. They tried calming me down but it would not work. Others got involved and there was no way they were getting me out without any violence, they would have to restrain me and escort me off the premises but they knew I would be back. I have to admit it was getting pretty ugly then my manager said, "Ok OK, you can have a copy, but you can't give this to your solicitor. It's only minutes of a meeting and this is only a draft." I agreed and he went off to get my copy done.

I left the office and went straight to the shop and bought an A4 envelope and some stamps. Of course I was going to send it to my solicitor and they knew it; I was not stupid. So there you have it, I have a solicitor who has not done a thing, their solicitor who had not done a thing also and here was there report saying the driver was right and we were wrong and we made mistakes. Open and shut case my dear Watson, put the kettle on and let's have a cuppa and let us wait for the cheque. Well no, not exactly.

A date came to court where the other side (as they will now be called) had to put up their objections to my complaint. Basically we had a list of health and safety measures that had not been adhered to, also my injuries to take into consideration, some loss of earnings, but not much as at this point as I was still on full pay. They had 28 days to respond to say whether they agreed or disagreed. The 28 days came and went and they did not respond so I rang Henrietta to find out what was going on.

"Well they have not responded which means they have admitted all liability in this case."

"So we have won the court case?" I asked in shock and amazement.

"Well yes, so all that need to be done now is to work out your damages and any loss of earnings and we can then put to them a schedule of losses. They then work out their schedule of loss and then we chisel it down and come to some sort of agreement."

"Wow, ok," I am in shock, is it really that easy? "So what now?"

"Well you will see a psychiatrist from both sides and a neurologist from both sides and they will meet and discuss your case and give us a prognosis and from this we can work out values."

Great I thought, a few medical appointments and we can put all this behind us and move on. I was extremely low at this point as I still had not had much in the way of treatment.

The appointments for the court case just seemed to take forever. I kept chasing Henrietta but she just didn't return my calls. In the end I got so sick of it I just emailed her instead. This was to become a huge mistake for me. I was deteriorating so bad at this point that I demanded she answer immediately. Why didn't she? I knew she would get my emails but then she would not respond. I became obsessed about getting this damn claim behind me. I did not believe for one minute that a cheque was going to cure my depression but I felt that it was an additional stress that I could do without. Suing someone is a very cold and a slow process. Everything is suited to the solicitors. Let's face it, who writes the laws? Solicitors, so who are they going to make sure comes out on top no matter if they win or lose? Solicitors of course. They aren't stupid after all. Here is a job where you have to follow rules created by yourself and you are paid by the hour. I mean come on, it's fucking heaven, a way to print your own money no matter if you win or lose. The thing with solicitors and barristers everything is either black or white, right or wrong or lawful and unlawful. There is no emotion involved whatsoever. On one hand this is good as you cannot expect them to be emotionally involved with their clients, but when you are down and suffering from depression, you start to feel like a number again. They get your file out, open it, ring you or write to you, then close it and work their way onto the next file. It's a sad fact of life, but your life is in their hands and they do not even know who the hell you are.

So I have won my case, surely the finishing line is ahead of us? Well as I said it's quite slow. It was six months before I had my appointment with the psychiatrist who would be presenting his findings on our behalf. He was an interesting man, in fact quite funny, he was as mad as a hatter himself. He was Indian, middle aged but had the most posh accent I had ever heard. He spoke as if he was in an Agatha Christie book. For this book I shall call him Dr A. We called him this in meetings that were yet to come as none of us could actually spell or pronounce his surname. He had a list of 30 or so questions to ask me and he did ask me but I never answered. Not because I didn't want to, but because he answered them for me. I would sit opposite him and away he would go.

"So tell me old boy, how is your sleep? Dreadful dreadful dreadful I bet, hardly sleep a wink does one? Mmmm mmm and your diet? Dreadful I bet, not eating, I know I know, hmmmm hmmmm." Each time he would write down the answer he had just given himself. I really did not need to be there. "So talk me through a normal day, up early I bet, feeling tired, watching TV, neglecting yourself and then terrible moods and the feeling of neglect, hmmmm hmmmmm yes I know I know. Do you still dream about the horrific crash? Of course you do, why am I asking? It keeps you awake all night, constantly playing the scenario over and over in your head. The explosion, the sounds, the pain it must be awful." Wow this guy was good. Either everything I was suffering he had guessed right, or it must happen to everyone in this situation, or he was just writing down all the things that were in my best interest when it would come to court. I left him wondering if I looked more ill than I suspected but as I was to find out, it's something called the court case game. It really is a game as well.

Let's look at this court case in the cold light of day. I have been injured, got a mental condition and then been treated like shit by my company. I am angry, I am depressed and feel like my whole life has been ruined. So the case now becomes the only way that I can inflict any pain on them whatsoever. In reality it's not pain at all. It's just a cheque from their insurance company, but it's a way for me to fight back, my only way. So what do I want? Money, and as much as I can. Now from the other side's point of view they have admitted liability and now it's all about damage limitation. They want to pay out as little as possible and the only way they can do this is to say I am not as ill as the psychiatrists say and everything will be ok once I have my treatment. That's the treatment they cancelled on me twice, but that is neither here nor there. So it becomes a game of wits and who has the strongest nerve. We aim high, they aim low and somewhere in the middle we come to some sort of settlement without it going to court. So over the next three years, yes in fact it was three and a half years from winning my case, which means the other side admitting it was their fault, I had to jump through so many hoops and attend appointment after appointment. There are two reasons for this. One, because they will not agree any figure until both sides agree a future prognosis, both psychiatrists, neurologists and as it turned out after I got sacked, employment consultants all had to write reports about my future. It was not until they all found common ground that we could progress. So my psychiatrist is telling everyone I am about to top myself, their psychiatrist could not see what all the fuss was about and basically said I had mild depression and I would be ok in three months, that was after a 15 minute consultation which after travelling two hours there he made me wait nearly 90 minutes past the appointment time, and then cut it short because he had tickets for something. It was becoming a joke. This game about my life and my future was a farce. It got to the point where you were almost believing stuff that was not true myself.

I mean, I knew the truth; I was ill, I have depression, anxiety and post-traumatic stress. These people had to write reports that best suited the people paying them, not what suited me. In the middle was me getting more and more frustrated as no one actually cared what I thought. If they said you should be like this in three months and you weren't they wanted to know why you weren't. Everything was waiting for deadlines and waiting for more appointments. One good thing was that all the neurologists agreed with each other. I was poked and prodded and they agreed to the paralysis down the side of my face and neck. Yet still every six months I had to go back and see them again to make sure they both agreed. They would do their tests and then six weeks later we would get a report with their findings and recommendations.

After a couple of years or so I met up with Henrietta. In fact it was a few weeks after they had sacked me. This changed the whole game completely because now the game had changed. Now we not only had to look into the future to work out what my health was going to do but also look into the future and work out exactly how much money I was going to earn and what sort of job I could get now I am no longer a train driver. Let's face it, if I got well again I would never be taken on as a train driver. They would not touch me with a barge pole and who could blame them? Hurtling along with hundreds of people on the back of the train and suddenly I have a manic episode, it wouldn't be good would it? So my career had well and truly gone. Also who would employ me? I would be 40 by the time all this had finished; too old and too ill to restart a new career, it was not looking good.

My solicitor reassured us and said do not worry, we will go to court this March and get it all sorted. I have worked out a schedule of losses for you and this is what we will be aiming for. This was in January, just two months I thought and it will be over, that would have been amazing. So we are in this meeting with Henrietta and she shows us this schedule of losses she has put together. It's about eight pages long and has loads of paragraphs and at the end of each one was a figure. Each one explained my future losses for that particular item, for example, future wages, money lost for future treatment, money lost for petrol to appointments the list seemed to go on and on. Then on the last page was a massive total. It was huge, I mean massive. I could not believe it. My wife and I queried it and she said it's all there in black and white, this is definitely what it works out to be. We could not believe it. I felt weird, elated on one hand but being dragged down with my depression by the other. It would be amazing if we could get that, it would change our lives forever.

So we were given the date, March 28th. The time to be there was 9.30am. We were going to meet our solicitor on the steps of the court just in case we needed to speak to her about any last minute details. It was completely unbelievable it would happen so quick, less than two years after the crash. Maybe this would be the point where I can put it all behind me? I would be free of my company and maybe start looking forward at last. The thing is once you have been treated so badly, your depression magnifies it a hundred times and so it becomes something that is very hard to deal with. All the stupid phone calls, the silly letters, all the appointments I had to keep going to. All the hoops I had to jump through just to get paid. It was not helping me at all. To be perfectly honest with you, the best thing that could have happened was for them to sack me as my expectations of them was now nonexistent. All I had to do was deal with being treated like damaged goods and move on. The court case however, meant I could have some payback. They would have to explain things in court, no more passing people from pillar to post. Now at last they would have to explain why they treated and neglected me so bad. At last I was going to have my day in court.

We heard nothing from my solicitor in the weeks leading up to the case but we accepted this, after all what had to be said was said and it was just a case of waiting for the date to come round. My wife had booked the day off to be with me all day; she knew it was going to be traumatic for me no matter what happens. So picture me the evening before, my wife and I am sitting there almost in silence. I have been sick, anxious for the last two days, I felt like crap. Then the telephone rings, its Henrietta. My wife has answered it. As she is talking to her she looks at me with absolute horror. I am gesturing to her to tell me what is wrong, but she is just on the phone still, listening and then says, "OK, I will tell him," and hangs up.

"What? What did she say, have they agreed to settle out of court? Tell me." Her face said it all really, I should have guessed.

"No, tomorrow's trial date has been cancelled. The judge is ill."

"What?"

"He is ill and it's been put back four weeks; it will now be the end of April."

A MAN DERAILED

I could not understand it, how can there only be one sodding judge to hear my case, what do they do when he goes on holiday for fuck's sakes? Close the court house down? I mean how ridiculous. Needless to say I was fuming. I was so angry and disappointed, so was my wife. All that anxiety leading up to this point and then being told that. Surely that must be nonsense, could it be true?

I was going to ring the court house to see if this was true, but my wife stopped me and said do not rock the boat, we just have to wait another four weeks. Another sodding four weeks.

My wife went back to work the next day and I was left to ponder what had gone on. My moods were dipping when I was not angry. This was during what I like to call my two gear period. One gear was anger and the other was depression. Up and angry and low and depressed. No middle ground and the court case was not helping. This no doubt made it impossible for my wife as she could not win. Over time she felt helpless as there was nothing she could do to help me. The thing is, she did the one thing she could have done to help me, it was the hardest and most incredible thing ever, she stuck by me.

This little story has a little twist. As we were told it would all be over at the end of March, we decided it would be good for us to go away for a holiday when it was all over. We decided to go to Malta and stay in a spa resort there. As we had been told by the wonderful Henrietta that that it would all be finished with at the end of March, we thought a holiday would be a good way to sort of celebrate and to kick start my recovery. The spa had everything you could expect from mud baths, salt water pools and every relaxing treatment you could imagine. We both needed it and both deserved it. We did not worry about money as we were assured that we would have the money in our bank accounts by then so we could go out there and have a completely stress free holiday. However, as the judge was now sick, it meant the court date was now moved to the day before we had booked to fly out. Looking back on it we were so stupid. We believed everything Henrietta said. If she said the judge was ill then he must be, if she says we will have our money by such a date we believed her. She had advised us all along this case from day one to this court date, why should we not believe what she had said? Even with my severe depression I thought of her as someone on my side, someone who would help us.

I had severe trust issues with people, especially the lies I was told about my treatment and how I would be well looked after by my management and then dumped in the bin like rubbish. It did not cross my mind that Henrietta would not be telling us the truth. So with the revised date it meant that we would now be going away with hardly any money. Like idiots we had spent quite a bit on the holiday and assumed we would use some of the money from the payment as spending money. A stress free holiday it was not going to be.

A MAN DERAILED

The four weeks went by like a snail; every day seemed to last forever. In the days coming up to the date I hoped the other side would settle out of court and that we did not need to go to court. Again my wife took a day off work and once again the night before the court date itself we got a call.

"Oh hi, it's Henrietta. I know this is not going to please you but the judge will not proceed with your case tomorrow. He wants more reports and an agreed long term prognosis for your condition. The good news is they have agreed to pay you an interim payment as I made them aware you are low on funds, so a cheque for £15,000 will be with you soon". I could not believe it. I have to be honest I cannot remember how the rest of the conversation went. Of course the money would help but I wanted all this over. I put the phone down and my mood dropped to what seemed an all time low and the very next day I have to fly to Malta. If only we did not book that damn holiday, we were so stupid, why did we think it would be ok? We were saved by my parents as they lent me some money and I swore blind I would pay them back as soon as the claim was settled. They gave me a cheque which meant waiting for a few days to clear. I flew out to Malta with just £15 in my account. We could not book any treatments until the second week when the cheque had cleared. Thankfully we booked an all inclusive holiday so all our food was in the price we had already paid. It was not a good holiday, which was a shame. I had been to Malta many times before and had seen this hotel being built and had always wanted to go there. We spent most of the time just walking around dazed, not believing what had happened.

We flew back after a fortnight, both feeling worse than we did before we went out. We knew it was going to be at least another year before this would be settled. On my return I had little money, no job, no treatment and I was losing all my hope. The cheque had not arrived so we were not very happy. I was angry and basically I was going to chew her arse off until I got the money through. I just did not care anymore.

Finally we got an envelope from them and I was hoping to find a cheque inside but all there was was a compliment slip from Henrietta and no cheque. I rang her immediately and told her; the envelope was slightly torn and it could have been taken out. I wanted her to get the cheque stopped. She took my call and said she would get replacements out to me as soon as possible. More time went by and nothing. I have to be honest we weren't in a bad financial way anymore as my parents had helped us with their cheque, but I wanted something that she had arranged to actually happen and go right. Every day I chased her. I didn't care; I became obsessed with this one piece of paper. Until I got it I would not rest. It's how the depression makes you, you will not lie down anymore and let others walk over you. My anger had kicked in and it would not go away until I got what I wanted. I guess I was like a huge child but I didn't care, I had been promised so much in the past two years and nothing had happened. Now I was going to fight for everything and make sure I got what was coming to me. I must have stressed Henrietta out of her mind, I did not care, but it worked. I then got a cheque in the post for the full amount and immediately paid it into my account. I did not notice at the time but the cheque was a hand written cheque from a normal savings account. It came from the name of Simon Harrison. Even at the time I thought it was a bit strange, but wanted the money in my account, so I paid it in. So now I got the money in the bank and now to get these damn appointments arranged.

I chased Henrietta everyday on the phone to make the appointments quickly. They never seemed to happen, it was so frustrating. It got to the point where she just ignored my calls, ignored my emails and would not respond to my letters. She had told me that case would be settled and it wasn't. I suddenly started thinking, what else was she not telling me?

Then one day I rang her office to pester her again. The receptionist answered the phone and I asked for her. "Oh I am sorry sir, she does not work here anymore, is there anyone else here who can help you?"

She had left, did not say a word, so I asked who would now be dealing with my case and she did not know. Actually it took over a week before anyone else contacted us and said they were aware of the case and someone was now dealing with it. My new solicitor was called Alison, she called me and introduced herself and said it may be a good idea if we met up and discussed the case. My mind started swirling around with all the weird things that happened with Henrietta and I knew there was something not quite right. Alison was treating me as if I was some sort of major case and that there was nothing she would not do to get us across the finish line and make sure it would be the right result for me. Suddenly I was important, but why? I was on the phone with Alison and we seemed to be going over old ground as if she was filling in the blanks, seemed strange. So I then asked, "Why did Henrietta leave?"

"Well, we have just relocated to a new office and she did not want to commute, so she left."

"Strange," I replied, "I would have thought she may have mentioned it, I assumed she knew for some time?"

"Oh, yes it was planned to merge these offices months ago." So why had she not mentioned it before, I was somewhat confused. My brain wanted to know more, but I knew Alison would not be comfortable talking about another colleague especially if it meant talking about them in a negative light. They are like doctors, will never say another doctor has made a mistake or did something wrong, always covering for each other.

"So why are we going over all these old appointments and conversations from the past?" I asked.

"Well I am afraid Henrietta did not update your file

that well before she left, so I just want to make sure all is as it's meant to be."

"But you are asking me about things that happened over a year ago. That's hardly recent is it?" There was silence. It was then I knew something was not right.

"Alison, can you tell me, how long had Henrietta been a solicitor?" She must have been new and made elementary mistakes. I started thinking she was as crap as I thought and they sacked her. Then, the bombshell, I did not see this one coming at all.

Alison replied, "Solicitor? No, she was not solicitor, she was just a paralegal. She maintained files and arranged appointments, that sort of thing. Why did you think she was a solicitor?" She was not a fucking solicitor, so for two and half years I had had my case dealt with by someone completely unqualified. She was just admin.

"So what solicitor has been dealing with my case?" I asked, in a rather worried tone.

"Erm well I am now, look Mr. Holmes, everything is fine with your case. We are moving on as per the court schedule and everything is fine." She tried to reassure me.

"What court schedule? But what about the two court dates we had in March and April? What were they supposed to be about?" I could feel the anger boiling; I remained as controlled as I could, as I wanted to know the truth.

"They were not trial dates, we haven't had any of those. They are just telephone calls with the court to update them with the progress of the case, nothing other than that."

"But she said they were trial dates, my wife took days off work to attend and you are now saying they were not trial dates. You mean the judge was not sick?"

"Sick?" she seemed surprised "No of course not, who on earth told you that?"

So basically for two years someone pretending to be a solicitor dealt with my case. As soon as I heard this I requested copies of all my files so my wife could go through them and see what was said. Was it all in my mind? Did I imagine it? I mean, surely I could not have got it so wrong, or surely I could not have had a sodding administrator dealing with my case. The files arrived, and then I realised why Alison was trying to fill in the blanks. It was because Henrietta had erased all records of our conversations and emails for the last six months. For some reason she had been telling me lie upon lie; I just could not believe it.

I then complained and had to deal with the most obnoxious arsehole I have ever had the misfortune to deal with in my life. I am so tempted to leave her real name in this book but I suppose I should not. So we shall call her Jenny. I told her about all the lies that Henrietta had told me, I had also found out by this point that the schedule of loss was totally unusable in court and would have to be re-done. Her response was as follows:

"Well I do not see anything in the files to back what you are saying. If it is not there it was not said." So in other words I was lying, I was making it all up, the reason why it was not there was because large chunks of my file had been shredded. All through the file there is a reasonable amount of information being put in every month, but the last six months of when Henrietta worked there had gone. Jenny did not see this as unusual. More arse covering by the solicitors. Why did I expect that she would help me? All this was happening during my lowest periods and how the hell I got through it I will never know.

It was then discovered that Henrietta not only deleted my file, she actually scanned my signature and made fake letters from myself placing them in the file. None of them had an original signature on as they were all scanned. One of these letters gave permission for the £15,000 cheque being paid to me to be signed over to a Henrietta Harrison. This was the cheque I waited ages for; she had made them pay it out to her. Harrison was her married name and she worked there under her maiden name. At first it looked like she had committed forgery to obtain money from me, but then it became apparent that they had paid me the money from her own account to make sure I got the money and then forged the letter to pay herself back. It was incredible. Why would she do this? Looking back, I guess it was because I became such a bastard towards her, she knew I was onto her not doing things right and by covering her tracks she got herself deeper and deeper into trouble. It is no wonder she left. So when all this forgery and fake letters in my file came to light, Jenny was a little bit different to me on the telephone. She rang me and I simply said, "Sorry Jenny, I want everything in writing from you and your company from now on. If it is not written down, it has not been said." This did not go down too well but I didn't trust anyone anymore, why should I? The police were called and Henrietta was just given a warning by the police and no further action had been taken. It appears she was having some sort of breakdown and my case was the one that suffered because of it. Obviously I was not the only one with a mental health problem dealing with my case. Also she was never supervised during all this time as no one else knew my case existed.

My wife scanned the so-called solicitor files and found 52 mistakes ranging from missing emails I had sent and she had replied right up to forged letters that I had never ever written myself. I complained to the Law Society and they did bugger all and said, "Yes they have really screwed up your case, but not much we can do." We put our case to the director of the solicitors and he was a complete prick. Like all solicitors he would not give me a straight answer to any of our complaints. After a lot of letters going back and forth it was obvious that I did not trust them and they felt it would be best if I went to another firm, which I did. Once again we had been dropped by a company that had screwed up and its only way out was to get rid of me.

So two years after all that nonsense, yes two years, during that time I had loads and loads of appointments and more and more reports, we were finally coming to the end. An additional report was needed as we drew closer to the end of the proceedings, it was an employment report. This meant I had to be evaluated for any other types of work I could do. The report for my side of the case took twenty minutes and the guy basically said, "Don't worry, I know what to write that will be good for your case." and abruptly left. The employment report for the other side however, was completely different. It meant yet another trip up to London. I was finding this harder and harder to do. It was not so much the train journey, it was the tube. Always full of people being trucked around like cattle, always too hot and always delayed I hated it. I braved the tubes and trains nevertheless. When I got to the correct street the heavens opened and I got completely saturated I was so close to just turning around and heading home.

I found the office and in I went. I was greeted by a lady very formally dressed and said that a Dr Roberts will be with me shortly. I was pre warned beforehand that Dr Roberts was a top class consultant and that he was wheelchair bound and running a very successful business. Then I heard the electric motors of his chair and Dr Roberts entered. He introduced himself and manoeuvred his chair behind the desk. All he could move was his right hand that controlled the joystick for his chair. I was not sure whether I should shake his hand or not so I did; it felt limp and lifeless but he seemed pleased that I was not affected by his disability and on we went.

I was then asked to answer what seemed like hundreds of questions. It was basically a psychometric test. Actually two tests. The first was to acquire what skills I had and the second to ask me what I really wanted to do. The questions would come up on a laptop and I had to pick one of five answers: dislike a lot, dislike, no preference, like and like a lot. It took an hour to get through them and then his assistant hit a button and a long list of jobs would be there for me to see. The screen went blank and then the jobs that I was suited to and fell into my likeable categories appeared. Number one on the list was, wait for it, DENTAL NURSE, number 2, AROMATHERAPIST, and number 3 was landscape gardener. These answers would make his report look stupid so he started to ask me to change some of my answers and be more flexible but I refused. I answered the questions truthfully and I was not going to change them for anyone. It is not like I could have manipulated the answers as I did not have a clue how it worked. I left his office with visions of myself in a dental nurse's outfit and to be honest it did not look too good. I know I can knock teeth out but I do not think that was what his program meant when it associated me with such a job.

A MAN DERAILED

So finally we had all the reports in. The psychiatrists agreed I was depressed and had a good chance of getting better, but did not know when. The neurologists agreed I had mild nerve damage down the left side of my head and face; it may go it may not, who knows? Certainly not them. The employment consultants agreed I would work again, but did not know when and what doing. Funny enough, dental nurse was not in the report when it was sent it, funny that.

So off you go to your barrister, oh yes, I had a barrister, and like all barristers they believe they are God and we should all bow down before them and accept every word they say to be the gospel truth. I know he earns more than God. When I got my files from the solicitors to investigate all the lies, I saw copies of invoices for over £700 per hour to prepare my reports etc. Nice work if you can get it. It was explained to me that after four and a half years since my crash and then three years after I actually won my court case, it was finally going to be settled. My barrister told me it would be very doubtful if it went to court at all and he was sure they would settle before the court date itself. Once again it was set for 28th March. I was not sure if that was a good omen or not. There was one last meeting to have before the trial date and that was called a settlement conference. We met in the other side's chambers and we all sat in two different rooms with the barristers meeting in the hall way outside the doors. They did this so we could not hear what was being said, but we heard every word. My life was being decided in a corridor by two very pompous arseholes and I could not do a thing about it. Needless to say they did not offer enough and my barrister advised me I would get more going to trial so off I went home and waited for the trial date. I was really nervous about the whole thing; I was worried about losing my temper in the court room if anyone from the other side said anything bad about me. I knew I would bite and would not be able to hold my tongue. I just did not want anything to screw it up. I know I would look mad in court and the judge would see that, but I did not want to be held in contempt, how the hell was I going to control my temper?

Then out of the blue I got a call from solicitor saying the other side had made an offer and, to be honest, it was about what I would get in court, what did I want to do? It was a tough choice but I would have done anything not have this stress on my shoulders any longer, so we accepted. It was quite an anticlimax to be honest, less than a week later we got the cheque in the post. I held it in my hand with the compliment slip. I had always thought I would jump up and down with joy, go and travel around the world, splash out on clothes and cars. I showed my wife, she gave me a hug and I said, "I better go and pay it in to the bank." My depression was still there; it did not matter how much money that cheque was for I would not be able to feel joy or elation. All that had happened was that one large stressful scenario had come to an end. Now the real fight of getting better and getting my life back in some sort of order would begin.

A MAN DERAILED

Chapter 8 - Hello, my name's Paul, and it's been six weeks since my last kebab . . .

Self harm is something very hard for others to understand. It seemed to be something others would do and had no place in my ever decreasing depressed world. I would meet others in group therapy with huge chunks of flesh cut or scraped from their arms. They had long gotten over trying to cover the scars; it was as if they wore them like army stripes saying, this is who I am so deal with it. Others would never speak of it, still ashamed, as they knew that no matter how much they talked about it no one would really understand why they did it unless they had done it themselves.

One day, as we sat in the group therapy session, it was noticed by the therapist that one of the girls had fresh wounds along the inside of her forearm. In fact we all noticed. Eyebrows were raised but no one said a word. You could see that every one of us wanted to ask, "Why do you do this?"

Thankfully the session started and we sat there with our cappuccinos, the smell of coffee filling the room, as did the wonderful sunlight that shone through some of the biggest windows I have ever seen. By noon it was like an oven in there and we all moved around the room avoiding the sunlight shining in our eyes like a bunch of manic depressive vampires. Today was no different. Jane, our therapist for today, welcomed us and informed us that today we were going to continue our cognitive behaviour therapy. This usually meant asking each of us in turn about something that had happened to us that got us down and then how we dealt with it. It was always awkward as she picked on you at random to start and whoever she chose looked like a deer in headlights. This time she started with Amy. She has fresh cuts healing along her arm, a skimpy vest top on so you really could not miss them.

"So Amy, can we start with you today?" The room went quiet, and all eyes focused on her. "Why don't you tell us about how you challenged any negative thoughts, just like we discussed last week?" Amy sat upright in her seat and leant forward. She then folded her arms as if to either hide the cuts or put a barrier up between us and her.

"Well, I had a row with my mum about money." Her voice was all timid and quiet. "She still thinks I am going to go and buy drugs so she only gives me a ten pound note, so once I buy the cigarettes I barely have a fiver to do anything else."

"So how did this make you feel?" asked Jane.

"Well bloody angry, I have not done any drugs for months and she knows that. She still doesn't trust me."

"So what did you do?" At this point we all expected her to describe how she got a knife and started to cut herself, slicing herself as if to show her mother how she was hurting her, or something along those lines.

A MAN DERAILED

"Well we rowed about it, and then we sat down and discussed it more. I then realised that my mum did not want me to go back to drugs as she was so worried. She cried and told me how much she loved me and we hugged." She seemed to relax, having told her story, and then added, "I thought my mum was trying to punish me but she is just protecting me and I challenged my negative thoughts and realised I would do the same if it was my daughter."

"Well that's excellent Amy, well done . . . who is next?" The other seven of us were truly disappointed. One by one we rattled off our stories and soon we were heading for yet another cappuccino break and a chance for the smokers to cover the footpaths with yet more butt ends. As we queued for our drinks Adam, a man in his late fifties, turned to Amy and said, "I am really sorry Amy, need to ask, why do you do that?" He pointed at her arms. As cool as anything she looked at him and said, "Have you ever just felt nothing? I mean nothing whatsoever, no depression, no happiness, no emotion whatsoever?"

"I don't think so," he replied.

"You would know if you did, well I get that, and I do this so I feel something, so I know I am alive."

I remember sitting there for the rest of the day and when I got home thinking what this nothingness felt like, something that could make you harm yourself. I just still could not understand it.

So what sort of person harms themselves? Well, I did.

So when I realised what I was doing it was a huge shock as I never realised I was doing it. I did it for so long that my body changed: it ached, it hurt every time I walked or got out of bed; every movement became a huge struggle. In fact I could not even tie my shoelaces as I hurt my body so much. I did not use a knife or any other weapon come to think of it. I used food.

Before the crash I was a keen cook. I loved to cook and create recipes from scratch, spending hours cooking splendid meals and desserts for my wife and I to consume on the evenings that I wasn't working. After the crash I just did not want to cook. The sheer enjoyment of creating dish after dish, allowing the aromas to fill the kitchen and dining room just gave me no pleasure at all. The takeaway and delivery leaflets that came through the letter box became my best friend. They all advertised curries, kebabs, chicken and chips and Chinese food. All this could be cooked for you, delivered to you and all you had to do was unwrap it and shovel it down your throat without any thought whatsoever. The problem was my illness caused anxiety so bad in myself that I could not even ring up for it to be delivered or I would not answer the door to pay for it and bring the food inside. I was always anxious about making the call. I would sit there from 5.30 pm looking at the phone knowing all I had to do was ring them, give them my address, tell them what I want and then wait. My anxiety was so bad I could not do this simple task. I had to wait for my wife to get in to make the call to order the food. She also had to answer the door and pay for it while I hid in the front room. Also by this point I was totally starving, I could not eat all day as I did not have anything in the house and was too ill to go out and get groceries. My wife would leave at 6.45 am to go to work and would be home at 6.30 pm after her commute up to London. She did not want the takeaways but I would be so insistent that we have them, almost as if my life depended on them. Sometimes she would cook, but making her cook after a 12 hour day at work, while I had been at home all day doing absolutely nothing, used to make me feel so guilty. My guilt also resulted in my mood lowering further, so to make me feel better we would order a takeaway.

So this meant my day was split in two: the daytime where I was hungry all day and the night when I was bursting at the gills due to eating excess takeaways. In the daytime I did not feel worthy of eating. I was alone all the time, no one to talk to, no one wanting to understand how I felt. I felt worthless. I started to hold food back from myself to punish myself. I would not eat or drink. I became dehydrated, incredibly hungry and started to feel pains in my stomach as well as lots of rumbling noises. During the day I became weak, always so tired as I had no energy to do anything. My thoughts darkened and as time went on I thought I was nothing more than a worthless piece of shit. Why should anyone want to talk to me or want to be with me? Who can blame them for turning their backs on me when I needed them most? I am nothing, I am better off dead. These thoughts are quite reasonable at the time, which looking back is quite scary. Then I had my night-time thoughts. My wife had come home from work and I had done absolutely nothing to clean the place; no washing up, no hoovering, no cooking etc. etc. The day had flown by in a black cloud of my own self-pity and self-hatred. I could see on her face how hard this was becoming for her. She would smile and say, "Don't worry, we will do the house work at the weekend. Now shall I sort out dinner?" She would order our takeaway, as usual I would order too much for myself, and we would wait for it to turn up. As she described her day in full, I would hear about all these different people she had to deal with, all this work she had to do and all the problems she would have to solve. I just sat there listening. I had nothing to say as I had not done a thing. This is one of the hard things when trying to socialise with others; if you do nothing all day what have you got to talk about? It's just easier not to socialise. In fact with depression it is far easier to do nothing then try to do something. That's the problem.

As the door bell rang I would dive into the front room and wait for her to pay and bring the food in. By this point in the day I would be salivating. The pains in my growing stomach were so great and lack of fluids meant severe headaches. Once the food was unwrapped and placed onto plates we would sit in front of the television and I would eat as if I had only a few minutes to complete my meal. One hand holding the plate the other shovelling in large chunks of kebab meat down my throat, kidding myself the salad part was healthy so it was all ok to do this. As my stomach became full I continued to eat more, like french fries and even the rest of my wife's food. My stomach knew it was full but the pain it felt as I shovelled more and more food down it made me feel I was punishing myself in the correct manner. I had failed my wife all day by doing nothing around the house and now I was being punished for eating a great big plate of grease and fat. I could have cooked something nice and light but my addiction to this type of eating just pushed all those thoughts out of my head and I just craved takeaway. Eventually money dictated that the meal of choice was doner kebabs with large fries. It was a simple decision really as a Chinese or Indian meal would cost twenty pounds and the kebabs cost under ten pounds. This would happen three or four times a week. I would have eaten it every day if my wife did not intervene. In fact it got so bad that the takeaway shop I used must have had caller display on their telephone as after time my wife did not even have to ask for anything or indeed give an address. She would ring and they would answer, "Hello, kebab shop, 1 extra large doner with chilli sauce, one small shish no chili sauce and a large portion of chips?"

"Erm, yes, thanks, goodbye." my wife would embarrassingly answer.

Eating the kebab was no pleasure whatsoever. Let's face it, a doner kebab is something you eat when you are pissed out of your brain on 10 pints of lager and the Indian restaurant won't let you in. I swallowed every greasy mouthful without thought, just stared at the television, chewing, swallowing and waiting for the pain in the stomach.

At first there was tightness in my belly and then, as the last mouthfuls of food were swallowed, the feeling became almost painful. I sweated and was almost out of breath from all the food I had eaten. In my mind the pain felt right. It was punishment for failing in life, for becoming weak, for allowing myself to turn into this big fat piece of crap that no one could possibly love and want to be with. The more I hated myself, the more I punished myself with food. The worse I felt, the unhealthier I felt, the more I felt I failed so more punishment was needed. Yet another vicious circle that had consumed me

This was a vicious circle that, if continued, would kill me. I was committing suicide slowly. The signs of my self-harm were not scars down my forearm but huge rolls of fat that grew around my waist; my legs that became sore as I walked, not just the aching of the knees and hips, the skin of my inner thighs rubbing, causing red rashes that seemed to burn as I walked normally. The rolls of fat stopped me from putting on socks. I was completely out of breath after getting to the top of my 13 step flight of stairs in my house. I sweated almost all the time, and not just because of the medication. Family had commented on how they were concerned about my weight. The black dog in my head lied to me. It told me they didn't care, they were just getting at me again and what the hell do they know? They cannot feel what I am feeling, they just think I am a worthless piece of crap and they should fuck off and leave me alone.

The symptoms got worse. I ate more and more kebabs. My heart pounded as if trying to push itself out of my chest if I went out walking at all. I needed something to break this vicious circle, I needed anything to make me see what the hell I was doing to myself

One of the problems I had was that I very rarely left the house. This meant I did not need clothing. A pair of shorts or sweat pants were all I needed and maybe a tee shirt just to lounge around the house. I never answered the door bell, so no one would ever see me, so I really didn't care how I looked. Getting through the day became physically more difficult and my mental state deteriorated.

Then one day I was asked by my employers to go to a medical in London. They were still paying me sick pay so every now and then would send me on this horrific jaunt, on a train, a tube and long walk to be examined by a doctor from the occupational health. I hated to travel by train. The explosion and aftereffects were still very fresh in my mind, so my anxiety shot through the roof knowing I would have to travel on the train. I had to force myself to go otherwise they would stop my pay. Ironically this appointment played a huge part in breaking the kebab cycle.

I got up in the morning, showered and then started

to look for clothes to travel up to London in. I got some jeans and a shirt and went to put them on but they didn't fit. I don't mean I could not just do the button up, I mean I could not even get my legs in them. The tee shirt looked like it had been spray painted on so tight and uncomfortable, there was no way I could wear it. I went through all sorts of trousers, tee shirts and shirts and nothing fitted. I had outgrown them all. Normally I would go into myself and feel guilty and self hatred and the circle would continue, but I had a train to catch to get to this medical, but what was I going to bloody wear? In the end I put on my sweat pants, the old baggy tee shirt I always wore and training shoes. I got my railway pass and some money and off I went. It was a hot summery day, late July. It was weird as for the first time ages I felt the sun and wind on my face; I became really conscious of it, it actually felt nice. Then all of a sudden, as I walked to the train station, both my ankles started to hurt and began to seize up. I started limping and every step became a huge effort as I tried to continue through the pain barrier.

I had to stop and sit on someone's front garden wall. There were old biddies walking past me with their shopping trolleys, mums pushing their prams and I was a huge slob sitting in pain on a wall with a waterfall of sweat pouring down my forehead. In fact already my clothing was saturated. I never made it to the appointment; I rang from my mobile phone and told them I was too ill. Thankfully they agreed another date. I made it home and collapsed on the sofa, my heart pounding and my shortness of breath scared the living daylights out of me. I had always imagined if this had happened I would be grateful; I had just wanted to die and not suffer this torment anymore. However, I was scared, my own mortality stared me in the face for the second time in my life. The first time was not my fault but this second time was totally my own doing. I had to change, I had to stop. My ankles and knees were like concrete and I could not do the most basic of tasks. I was 37 for God's sakes.

The weekend came and my wife decided we both should go into town, if only for a little while. We drove to the car park and gingerly walked into the high street. As we walked into Boots the chemist to buy some toiletries my wife spotted the weighing scales. I was 20 stones at the time of my crash. I had always been a big guy, but I had been fit with weights and rugby so it was never a problem. She ushered me over to it and said "Come on, let's see how much weight you have put on and then we will work together to lose it." I put in my money and stepped on. The digital display flickered backwards and forwards and then stuck on a figure, which it printed out for me: 27 st 11 lb.

Myself harming eating disorder had made me gain nearly 8 stone. A wave of embarrassment hit me. I was completely stunned. In fact I was speechless. I could not believe it; surely it could not be right? My knees however said it was right and I needed to stop this stupid binge eating and starvation lifestyle.

Another problem related to the fast food addiction

and punishing myself was alcohol. Even though the excess weight and no food during the day made me dead tired I still could not sleep at night. I would lie there with a full stomach and feel sick. I was not comfortable at all. Then I discovered that drinking large quantities of beer before bed seemed to make me feel more empty and more comfortable. I could drink eight cans of beer quite easily and not think a thing of it. I would not say I enjoyed the drinking, but it was the only time I felt anywhere near relaxed and able to close my eyes and sleep. Sometimes after a good drink I could sleep for six hours. That's twice the amount I was normally sleeping. I just did not see the point in stopping. Having an off-licence dead opposite my house was not a good thing to have. I thought the guy was going to open up an account for me. I kept the place opened for months. Then the great shock of knowing I had put on eight stones in weight because of my eating and drinking habits shocked me. I knew if I wanted to sleep I either had to exercise myself enough to knock me out or get sleeping tablets. I chose the latter as it seemed a lot easier but the morning after feeling was awful and stopped me from functioning during the day. I then knew I was either going to drop dead or I had to make huge changes in my life. I had to change my eating habits.

It took a while but slowly over time I ate yoghurt in the morning, anything solid I would throw up. As I became accustomed to the breakfasts I was not so hungry at lunch. I would eat some fruit and slowly over time my energy levels increased. My weight

A MAN DERAILED

remained high for some time but I stopped the increase, which was the most important thing to do. My state of mind slowly stopped wanting to punish myself. I found the two things to do to stop this were to not give it a reason to punish myself and also stop eating the crap takeaway in the evening. Thankfully this has happened and, as I write this, I am now vegetarian and I have never felt this good for a very long time. I pray it lasts forever.

Chapter 9 - I don't want the fucking vegetarian cannelloni.

By the time the court case was settled I had been vegetarian for two months. I ate my last fry up in a hotel on New Year's Day. As each bit of gristle and fat eased its way down my throat I mentally said goodbye to my meat eating days. The smell and texture of the fried black pudding almost gave me second thoughts but I was determined not to go back on my pledge to commit myself to vegetarianism. I even made sure I told people beforehand so I was not likely to go back on it, but why? I guess I actually wanted to do something good and worthwhile in my life, I wanted to do something that would help my mind and body be healthy.

Cutting dead animals out of my diet seemed like a good solution. Let's face it, we have not got a clue what they pump these poor animals with to make them grow quickly. Unless you buy from a farm that you can see all the conditions that the live stock live in then, then don't buy. I am not going to preach and say we should all be vegetarians as I believe we all have a choice of what we should and should not wish to eat. We are very lucky in this part of the world. We can walk into a supermarket and pick up almost anything we want. Even though as I type this there are concerns about the increase costs of basic foods and oil etc. you can still walk into a supermarket and buy a chicken ready to roast for under £3. Is £3 really worth the life of that bird? Well I do not think so. You may think differently and that's your choice.

So with the fry up gurgling in my guts on that fine sunny New Years Day, and yes it was a New Year's resolution, I started my on my path to vegetarianism. Vegetarianism, that's a long word isn't it? Incidentally, before I progress with my story, vegetarians do not eat seafood or fish. Got it? It's great when you tell someone that you are a vegetarian, you have some wonderful conversations like:

Me: "Hi, how are you? Oh did I tell I am a vegetarian?"

Other nameless person: "Oh my God, really? Oh, erm well, what do you eat then?"

Or

Me: "Hi, how are you, oh did I tell I am a vegetarian?"

Another nameless person: "So you eat fish then? You got to eat fish for your brain."

Or

Me: "Hi, how are you, oh did I tell I am a vegetarian?"

Yet another nameless person: "Oh you poor thing, how long have you been like that?"

Me: "Eh?"

I just nod, it's so much easier. I have had five years of people who were ignorant of depression, I just could not be bothered to explain vegetarianism. It really was not worth it.

The weird thing that happens when you start this new healthy eating style, as I like to call it, is that you spend all your time finding meat replacements. So you buy vegetarian sausages, burgers, pies, pasties and eat endless amounts of cheese, pasta and rice. In fact you eat everything except fruit and vegetables. Once you get into the swing of things and start eating more fruit and vegetables cooking becomes quite stimulating. You realise there are countless wonderful tasty items to buy and cook. I wish someone would tell that to restaurants. Usually most of them will have one very poor vegetarian option and it's usually vegetarian cannelloni. Always the same. Why can they not cook lovely dhal, Spanish omelet's, risotto, the list is endless. Of course when you go to a place and order your vegetarian cannelloni it's obviously the one frozen pack they have at the back of the freezer, then micro waved and then poured onto a plate with a bit of rocket laying there all limp. Why do chefs think that by placing rocket next to a piece of slop it will then turn the meal into an amazing looking dish? I have not got a clue. It always tastes the same; a very mild pissy cheese sauce with lumps of flat pasta floating on your plate. I wish they would try harder. You imagine the scenario in the kitchen. The chef pours out this beige slop in a bag. It's piping hot with green bits of spinach floating horrible on the surface. So with years of training behind him, learning how to make amazing desserts, soufflés and amazing sauces he comes up with a cunning plan. "I know, I will put a handful of rocket next to it."

His staff are amazed with his artistic skills. They place it on a tray and charge me fourteen quid for it. Thanks for that.

This change to my eating habits had two very desirable affects in my life and one or two not so desirable ones as well. Firstly I was waking up very hungry in the mornings. My evening meal had been burnt off during my sleep, I would wake up completely empty then walk down the stairs and meet my dear old friend the lovely cold glass of water and then I would actually want to eat breakfast. This would have been unheard of last year. I would not eat anything until 6 pm and wondered why I felt mentally and physically drained all day. Now I wake, I drink and I eat. I give my body the energy it needs to allow my brain to function. Bowls of cereal and milk with a nice cup of tea. I know it doesn't seem like much to shout about, but this was a huge thing for me to do. Not only did it help my mind to operate it also gave me the energy to actually physically do stuff. Eating the fruit and vegetables kept me hydrated and feeling alive inside. I didn't need pills; I needed apples, salad, avocados, melon, goats cheese, brown rice and chickpeas. I cut out as much caffeine as I could, but I tell you that's not as easy as you think.

The damn headaches you get by cutting out coffee and tea are pretty bad. Not quite like migraines but a dull ache in front of your head. No matter what painkillers you take it never really goes away. I hated them so much I had to give in. I cut down my coffee intake from around 10 cups a day down to 2. The headaches were not as bad after a certain amount of time. The amazing thing was, and this isn't rocket science, I actually started to sleep longer than three hours a night. The caffeine I had in my body made me irritable and moody, making my state of mind even worse than it should have been. The problem is, when you are depressed you do not care what you eat, drink or indeed how you feel. So you pour down the coffee and become addicted to the little bit of a buzz you get all day. Take away the coffee and no buzz. I tried decaf but, let's face it, that's like a party with no music so what is the point? So I stuck with my water and continued to eat fruit and vegetables till they came out of my ears.

So I felt hydrated, energised, less moody and full of wind. My God, how much wind can one person emit? I really got into the pulses in a big way. Lentils, chickpeas and other beans would be cooked in chillies, curries and dhal. Then maybe a dab of fresh yoghurt with some strawberries for dessert. Then, at about 3 am, I would awake as if someone was stabbing me from the inside. The huge wind pains would bend me over double. I had a toilet seat imprint on my arse. I never seemed to be off it. If I was off it, it was only to cook yet another bloody dinner. Well not bloody, but you know what I mean?

My wok became my best friend in the kitchen. Let's face it, when you have depression performing tasks that take ages is not very attractive. In fact you talk yourself into failing before you start and you just do not do it. Now a wok means fast, even its name is quick and easy to say: heat it up, cut up some fresh veg, some soya sauce and a few chillies and you have a wonderful meal. It takes only one or two minutes on a high heat. You swirl the veg around, just like they do on the TV. You have the all the hissing steam, the amazing smells of a Chinese restaurant right there in your own house. Wonderful meals in minutes. It was excellent for me as I had the concentration span of a goldfish, so long complex meals held no interest for me. I cooked everything for the last couple of Christmases and felt like committing mass murder at the end of them. Here was a way for me to cook stress free and very quickly. It worked; it still works.

The great thing in supermarkets is you can buy these stir fry packs, little sachets of sauces and stir fry noodles, so cooking using a wok is literally just pouring three packets of food into a hot wok, stirring it and then serving. I mean how good is that? I know it's lazy, but the alternative of yet another takeaway was not good and at this time of my life I was not ready to go back to following pages of recipe books, I just could not do it.

Of course you soon become bored with the same bloody stir fried meal every night, so I started to investigate other more interesting options. Bean curd, tofu and soya mince all fell into the equation so I started to cook bolognaise, chilli con carne and curries. They were all things that I had loved before I was ill and a vegetarian and now I was discovering that I could have these meals again with a meat substitute. I bought what seemed like hundreds of vegetarian and vegan cook books and slowly over the last few months learnt how to cook healthy meals that were tasty and quick. During my really bad days I hated cooking and this made me feel very low as I always cooked in our household. Not because my wife can't cook, but because I always loved cooking. I think cooking from scratch for others to enjoy is one of the greatest acts a person can do. You give them wonderful smells, amazing colours and mouth watering tastes and in return you always get complimented. Well let's face it, you are not going to criticize someone who is going to prepare your dessert are you? However, due to our disappearing friends and my complete lack of motivation to perform any tasks, dinner parties were soon becoming a thing of the past. It's very sad, but something I hope to put right in the future.

Over time, as I gained my confidence back at the stove, I started trying more varied recipes. That's when I fell in love with a falafel. I had never really eaten falafels before, and if I did it was only prepacked ones you just heat through in the oven. They were ok, but hardly memorable. I had bought a Middle Eastern vegan cook book and there was the recipe to make them from scratch. I got a tin of chick peas, garlic, cumin, parsley and coriander. You measure out the right amount with a bit of salt and pepper and blend them into a sort of paste. You then make little balls and deep fry them for about one minute. That's how quick it was. They tasted gorgeous. I was never a lover of chick peas; if I ever cooked them it would always be in some sort of strong curry sauce, but fresh falafels were a triumph. That's when I noticed that by performing these recipes I had to read books. That meant that my concentration span was increasing. Then I had to go to the shops to buy the ingredients, showing my motivation to leave the house had improved. Then I had to perform the task of cooking. So because of this diet change it seemed to stimulate my brain into working in a more positive way. This meant I made myself feel better because I was actually achieving stuff and making a contribution to home life that was actually positive; it was wonderful. At last my vicious circles were spinning the other way. I started to feel good and over time gain some self belief. Who would have thought a falafel could do all that huh?

Chapter 10 - John! You sadistic bastard . . .

With my claim settled it would have been easy to fly off and have loads of holidays and buy lots of material things that frankly I did not need. I knew this would not be a good idea. I needed to use the money to give me some security and maybe help my state of mind. Just because you get a cheque in the post it doesn't mean that your depression would fly out the window and allow you to carry on from where you left off. As I learnt, only if you spend wisely, can money bring you happiness, or should I say less depression? I knew that despite my newly found way of eating I was not really getting as healthy as I should be.

My moods were still all over the place but I was sleeping better and felt better. However this was ok if I was just staying indoors with nothing to do I needed something that was going to make me fit to return to society. Something that would give me self confidence, something that would help me feel good about myself, something that would make walking down the shops a breeze and not like climbing Everest. So what could this magic ingredient be? Well it certainly did not come in a child-proof bottle from the chemist. The first step was to rejoin the gym. The thing is, you do not need to go to the gym to exercise, you can walk the streets, use tins of beans as dumbbells or if you are mad enough, and I clearly wasn't, you could cycle in the streets. No matter what, I knew that I had to exercise. I also knew how easy it would be to join a gym and never go back again. When I exercised in the past I had always felt good afterwards, physically lighter, I would be more relaxed and a much nicer person to be around. I knew I had to do something so I joined. I got shown round the gym by a guy who looked liked he was the bass player from Busted. He was nice enough but seemed to be more interested in the ladies in Lycra pounding the treadmill. He showed me the forms, I filled them in, and then there was a little box at the bottom of the form asking me if I would be interested in a personal trainer. For some reason, I ticked it as yes, but I assumed it would be some sort of marketing ploy to see who would actually use one and thought nothing of it. Of course we would all love personal trainers, barking out orders and encouraging us to change our lives but, let's face it, it doesn't happen in the real world, does it?

So my forms all filled out, I was told I will get my membership card in a few days and said my goodbyes.

So, I am home, sitting in front of the computer, no doubt writing a little bit of this book and the phone rings. A very young sounding man on the other end of the phone introduces himself as John. He is a personal trainer from the gym and wanted to know if I wanted to book an appointment to talk to him and start a course of exercises with him? I was gobsmacked, I was shitting myself. I was bad enough with strangers as it was but to meet someone and show them how incredibly ill I was, well that would be almost impossible. I hate meeting new people, I usually hate them and they hate me. I panicked and remembered I was going to go to Cornwall for a couple of weeks and this gave me a legitimate reason to say no. I would be able to say no for now and I would ring him back, which of course I wouldn't.

While away in Cornwall I saw people surfing on the wonderful beaches of Perranporth. I saw people sailing and kite surfing; they were all fit, they were all healthy they were all happy. I stood there feeling like a pathetic fool who let life pass him by. Depression had gripped me and held me down for too long. I had used depression as an excuse for far too long. The stress and disappointment of being the lonely soul looking in from the outside had finally got to me. I needed to change, I needed a kick up the arse, I needed someone to grab my by the ears and shout, "For God sake, you are 40, you are over half way through your life, make a difference, take a chance, for fucks sakes be happy." Well maybe not ears, as I would not hear it, but you get my point.

I returned from Cornwall and despite having two weeks of rain, the fact that I had been out of my cage for two weeks had done me some good. As I was unpacking the suitcases and emptying the wash bags we had taken with us I thought about that voice of John on the phone. He seemed chirpy enough, maybe I should ring him? Two days went past and I still had not rung. I was still doing the same old routine which was bordering on nothing with the odd shopping trip thrown in here and there for good measure. Then two things happened: firstly, I got an envelope through the door and it contained my membership card from the gym. Secondly, the phone rang and on the other end was John. I was sweating like mad, I was nervous, here was just a phone call sending me into almost panic. How can I commit to an appointment that I will be petrified to keep? I mean, I could barely walk last year and here I am discussing an exercise regime. It was as if my good half of my brain took over the conversation while the depression dealt with all the physical aspects, the pounding chest, the sweating, the shakes and the fear. I hate the fear. It happens before almost everything I arrange, and nearly every time I go to something I wonder what the problem was. It's almost an anti climax. This would be different. I would have to wear shorts and a tee shirt and get onto machines that probably would not hold my weight. It would be an embarrassment. How the hell was I going to get through all this? My calm side of my brain managed to make an appointment. This calm side was a recent thing that had happened. I could not even remember the last time I was calm or together. I always felt that the desire to be well took over like a natural instinct; I knew this was what I had to do. So it was all set, I was going to have a personal trainer. Shit.

I did not sleep the night before the appointment. I was sitting downstairs at my usual time of 4 am with a cup of tea, worrying if this one cup of tea would give me stitch or cramps, or would I vomit? I mean I played rugby after six pints of Guinness once because their front row had not turned up and boy did I vomit during the game. It was handy as no one would tackle me due to the stains down my rugby top. I may have even scored however due to the half time three pints I cannot remember. Would I vomit after these cups of tea? As I waited for the time to come where I would have to leave I played every bad scenario in my head. I imagined falling backwards off the treadmills, my shorts splitting and my arse hanging out as I bend over to pick up some weights. I had gotten used to having wardrobe malfunctions since piling on all the weight.

Another legacy of my rugby days, apart from spewing up Guinness, was big thighs, steady girls. I used to play in the front row which means the fat ugly blokes at the front of the scrum who grab each other's testicles to bind to each other while contesting for the ball. To be a prop you not only had to be able to grab testicles but also hold up huge amounts of weight as you smashed into the other side's front row. This meant big thighs, lumps taken out of my forehead and a bad back. Of course my big thighs just got bigger and fatter as more and more weight piled on thanks to those bloody steroids, anti depressants and doing absolutely nothing from one day to the next. This meant my thighs rubbed when I walked so my trousers would last about two weeks after the crutch would wear out due to the intense rubbing and friction burns of my legs. Of course I would not always realise this and there have been many a

A MAN DERAILED

time I have been in the waiting room of some shrink or quack, innocently sitting there waiting to be called with my bollocks perched nicely between my legs being held by a bright pair of underpants. I had noticed it would never happen when I had underpants on the same colour as my trousers; I think it's called sod's law. So the reaction of someone sitting opposite me was usually an indication that the trousers had frayed and it was time to close my legs or cross them. Oh happy days.

Back to the gym. The really worse scenario was I did not know how fit I was. Well I knew I was not fit, but not how bad. Would I have a bloody heart attack? I mean that would be the cherry on the cake after finally mustering enough strength to get down there, get changed, walk into the packed gym, have a panic attack then drop dead. Just my fucking luck. Oh well, here goes.

I pulled up in the car park, walked over to the reception, handed my card over and in I went. My stomach was churning, like a washing machine on spin rinse. Round and round it went; I had a feeling my tea and I were going to be reacquainted. I dumped my bag and personal belongings in the locker room. I forgot how long it had been since I had seen naked men spraying the most god-awful deodorants all over the place. My eyes were stinging when I walked out but hey, I smelt good.

Then finally the moment I had been waiting for, I met John. A very young Greek Adonis of a chap who obviously works out and for some reason he could not stand still. We shook hands and introduced ourselves. Together we looked like a whippet trying to train a Saint Bernard.

"Right, let's head off to the office," and off he sprints. I expected him to say beep beep before he walked. So we sat in this office and he asked me what I want to achieve, well that was a tough question. I just wanted to go home, but that was not on the agenda. I knew I wanted to lose weight, get fitter but most importantly please please please improve my state of mind. I did not go too over board about my depression. In fact I felt I hid it quite well. I was not sure if it was the best thing to do. I mean, I was worried that if he asked me what was wrong and what did I want to fix, I would not stop talking for the whole hour. It's weird because when you have had so much therapy you start talking nonstop about yourself as if nothing else matters. In the real world you cannot do that. Other people do matter and, let's be honest, they do not want to hear the ins and outs of a duck's arse about your problems. I was there to work out.

Well, what can I say about John? He has got skills that I do not even think he realised he had. He was extremely friendly and put my mind at ease almost immediately. He is extremely young, 19 going on 20. I mean what does he know about life? He knows nothing, but I was not there to get a course on living a better life. I was there to get hot, sweaty and completely out of breath. He knows how to get people fit, after all that's what he trained to do, and he is fit and bursting with energy. I am sure in a million years' time when all the humans have died out, a spaceship will land, having been attracted by a beacon buried under ground. They will land their craft somewhere where Southend on Sea once stood, they will dig down exactly where their instruments had said the beacon was coming from. That beacon will have some crocodile clips attached to it and on the other end will be John's bollocks, that's how much energy he has. It's bloody endless.

Before I am let loose in the gym I get weighed, have my blood pressure taken and then my body mass index is worked out. This is so we can see the improvements as time goes on; assuming I was to return that was. As usual the scales only went up to 22 stones; they did not have the freak size that was required to give me the exact reading I required. Being a 4 xl and a 50 waist meant I was used to everything being far too small for me. Café chairs, cinema seats, even modern day cars needed the front seats in to get my legs in; it's a bloody nightmare. However I am making that right, hence why I am here with captain power balls. If some of that energy could rub off on me then I could be onto a winner. My blood pressure was surprisingly near normal, but of course my BMI number was the same as a walrus that had just eaten a double decker bus; it was not good, I knew that. Again that was why I was there. Having your own physical imperfection there in front of you in black and white could send me into a deep depression, even though it told me nothing new. It showed me how much this depression had damaged my health. My biggest fear was that it was not too far gone for me to get it back to some sort of normality. I mean I was looking at losing 10 stone. That's 140 pounds, that was nearly two Johns. Depression makes you believe nothing good will happen and I have to admit I thought I was wasting my time, but John said in a very fast but calm way, "Beep beep , no problem, that will go, we shall sort it out." He didn't really say beep beep, but he said something that was quite different to anything that I had heard before. He said WE. I was going to go the gym and not doing it alone. He was going to be the kick up the arse I really needed. OK, I was going to be paying for it, but it was from money I never had before. I was actually getting someone who was going to change my mental state of mind. He was quite oblivious to how ill I am or indeed was. I am not saying he did not care, but he was looking forward at what I could achieve if I put my mind to it and all I was doing was looking back at all the shit that was holding me back. I had to look at the page in his clip board and believe that over time these numbers of weight, inches, heart rates and blood pressure would get better every month. I had to look forward, and that was before I did any exercise. It was bloody working.

So we left the office and I sheepishly walked past a spinning class. This seemed to be a group of 30 people sitting on these exercise bikes all facing towards with a dominatrix in cycling shorts at the front. As the music blared out she screamed instructions at them. It was as if their lives depended on doing what she told them. Every one of them was covered in sweat, their legs pumping the pedals like mad and their faces all a wonderful beetroot colour. I did not envy them.

So, Beep Beep, on to the treadmill. I had to start a warm up; the machine started at a nice leisurely pace. Not too bad I thought. I can manage this, like walking down the beach. Of course this did not last; slowly he increased the speed. I held onto the handles for dear life. I pretended to be cool, but the fact that I could not talk as I walked made it quite clear I was getting warmed up rather nicely. I assumed after the treadmill we would go to all the other torture machines that line the gym, but oh no, we are going to do circuit training. I remember circuit training from my rugby days, it always seemed easy as it was just a load of leaps and squats with medicine balls or hand weights, however once you got half way round you really knew you had a work out going on.

He must have really hated me because boy, did he hurt me. I throw medicine balls onto the floor as hard as I can, making a huge booming sound echo all around the gym. Making one of those things bounce so you can catch it at waist height is bloody hard. Then some step work with dumbbells, then lunges and then the god awful plank. It's not just what you feel like when you do it, the plank is an exercise that is supposed to be good for your inner core muscles. They are called core muscles because when you exercise them you say "Core blimey that hurt." Sorry, crap joke. You lay face down on the floor and then lift your body off the floor just using your nose and toes. Ok, not your nose, but your elbows, but it might as well be your nose. As you lift up every muscle in your body screams, "For fucks sakes what you doing?" and then you collapse in a huge puddle of sweat on the floor. "OK Paul, just hold that for five seconds." Five seconds? Is he having a laugh? He must really hate me.

As the workouts progressed I felt as if John had been bullied at school buy a big fat bald guy with a goatee and this was his chance of revenge. He really put me through my paces. He would hand me a big metal ball with a handle on it and tell me to swing it between my legs and push my arms up in the air by just thrusting with my hips. It sounds easy enough, but after eight it's killing you; your arms ache, your back and your buttocks are almost going into spasm. Because you are thrusting with your hips, he would shout, "Shag the ball, that's it five more times, shag it hard." Sex was nowhere in my thoughts and the thought of my tackle hitting this metal ball really didn't do it for me. The step box or whatever it's called, that big grey and black box you just step on and off looks innocent but put it in John's hands and after two minutes you feel like you need a rope and tackle to get up it. I had to step on it and step off. That was quite easy and then he gave me these piddly little dumbbells, they were only five lbs each. I mean, come one, I know I can lift more than that. "Ok, as you step on the box I want you to perform a hand curl with the dumbbells and then step off, then change legs and do exactly the same thing." Is that it? I thought. So with my tiny matchstick weights in my hand I step on the box and do a hand curl and off again, after five I was warming up, by eight the dumbbells had miraculously turned into two Austin Minis and weighed a bloody ton. With every curl the weights got harder and harder to lift, each step seemed to become bigger and harder to do. "Are those weights too light for you? There are some heavier ones there if you need them."

"No no I am fine, these are fine." I would reply. I would be standing there like a pig fountain. Out of every pore in my skin, sweat would be squirting out like there was no tomorrow, and the way I felt I didn't think there would be a tomorrow. John was hurting me good. He did it with a smile, he knew how far to push me and would not hold back even if I said I had had enough. Each exercise he would spur me on shouting, "That's perfect. Just five more to go." It was always five more to go, never one or two. Always bloody five, but it pushed me on. You did not want to let him down or indeed more importantly yourself. John showed me that I could and still can push myself and start to change things around. Each time I left the gym I felt like I was on cloud nine, I was walking but could not feel my legs, not because of pain but because I felt so light; it was and is still today a truly amazing feeling. Each time I go my body is the important thing, my brain comes second. This time the side effects of working out dull the depression, and allow me to have energy and control of my life again. I had never believed this would ever happen again. I would leave the gym elated, drive home and sit down but, and it's a big but, I could not sit down; I wanted to do something. So I would tidy up, wash up, go to the shops and do the mundane things I had neglected for so long. I had energy, I wanted to do stuff. Of course this only lasts a couple of hours because about three hours later I am in bed having a nap. Then I would go to bed at night exhausted and actually have a deep sleep; a few times going through to 6 am, I mean that's like eight hours sleep; I mean, come on, eight fucking hours. Nearly five years to get back to that. It was a complete life change for me. Not only was I sleeping but I had energy and was eating at regular patterns during the day, my weight started to decrease and I started to feel better about myself. Did you hear that? I actually started to feel worthy of living, being in society, being a husband, a friend, a son or maybe a work colleague. I was beating this bloody depression. Could it be possible that I could control it rather than it me?

This was a huge turning point for me. I did not have any shrink or GP telling me what to do, no pills or potions or indeed no group therapy, just a regular trip to the gym.

So here I was making huge steps. I am vegetarian, working out regularly and generally feeling better about myself. The anxieties had seemed to have retreated somewhat and my anger problems seemed to take a back seat. I was and am calmer and dare I say it, happier?

A MAN DERAILED

So it took a young whippet of a man to show me that physically I can achieve whatever I want if I put the time and effort in. Maybe I just got lucky with meeting John or maybe all personal trainers are like him, I do not know. All I know is that it works and I am glad it has happened. I know you will be reading this John so cheers mate, see you next week.

Chapter 11 - The Domino Friends.

The one thing I have had to deal with over the past few years is people's total lack of understanding of what depression is all about. I have to admit I was, and sometimes even now, am not an easy person to be around, but you have to remember it is nothing personal. I guess unless you have suffered you will never truly understand. Of course I do not want to be alone, with hardly any social life, being cooped up indoors 24/7. The problem is the depression makes you feel totally unworthy of having a good life. You do not feel good enough to have people's friendship; you almost go as far as to destroy those bonds you have had in order to satisfy your own self worth. It is self-destruction, it is beyond my control and yet it is me that is doing it. I stopped ringing people because they never rang me first, so I believed they really did not care about me. When they did ring me to go out somewhere, I felt they were only asking me to go out of pity and, combined with my anxiety about leaving the house, I would not go.

I projected all my negativity on my friends and some family members, I made reasons not to see them and even contact them in any shape or form. The few times I did meet with people they had a complete lack of understanding of what I was going through, but of course they would, how could they understand? I guess when I had the crash I wanted everyone to drop everything and come to me, to constantly ask me how I was, to prove to me that they cared and gave a damn. Apart from my wife, no one did. The problem was that my damage from the crash was 99 per cent mental, that's the part you cannot see and the physical face part didn't bother them much so they didn't even mention it. The damage was invisible and still is.

At first you don't go around shouting to everyone, "Hey guys, I got depression and post-traumatic stress, how about we go for a meal some time?" You suppress it, you hide and try to get on in life. If I had a penny for every time I was told how much better I would be once I got back to work or to pull myself together and stop thinking about the past I would have a big bag of change. I was constantly being told to move on and starting planning the future. Get back in the saddle and all that sort of thing. The problem was I was petrified of leaving the house and had severe depression. I lacked any motivation to do anything about it. I assumed people came to you and helped because they cared, because they gave a damn, but I was wrong.

My long time friends, in all honestly, did not treat me any different. I just didn't feel I belonged anymore. The few times I did meet them I felt awkward and I did not act myself. We would usually go to pubs and drink quite bit, this made me more and introverted and I said less and less. I knew they sensed there was something wrong but, instead of coming up to me and asking me about it, they drew back. It was quite difficult to handle. Like an idiot I assumed they cared and would make an effort. The problem with depression is that you have high expectations of people. My expectations for my friends were too high quite quickly and over time one by one we lost contact. No sooner had I lost contact with one, it turned out the mobile number I had for another was out of date and on and on the changes happened without me knowing. I guess I pushed them a bit and they stepped back a lot. It really is quite sad and I truly regret it ever happened. The problem is I am always resentful of that. All they had to do was make one call or a text message, but nothing. Of course I could have done it myself and taken the initiative but I am afraid to say depression does not work like that. It seems to thrive on you being lonely, with no social life and feeling guilty for the all the comments I said in the past.

Though I did find out who my true friends are; they know who they are and I will not forget how they did stick by me and not topple over so easily like the others.

My advice to people who discover their friends or family have depression is quite simple. Hang on in there with them, they may say stupid things like, "leave me alone, I am not worth it," or, "What the hell do you care, you don't understand," and I am not going to say they don't mean it, because they do. You just have to accept it's an ill version of your friend or family member who is talking. Imagine feeling you are worthless or you are so low in mood you would rather be dead, and I do not mean that in an off the cuff type statement to make, I mean really dead. That person sees no future, no reason to live for, no joy, no excitement, doesn't feel love and cannot give it either. He hasn't chosen to be like that; these are symptoms you have with depression. If I smashed a brick over your head and you lost your sight, how would you feel if someone said, "pull yourself together" or, "come on, move on, what's wrong with you?" You would consider them a very insensitive bastard. I mean how can you say that to someone who has gone blind? I appreciate that the symptoms must be horrid if you go blind but we try and make allowances for them, we even help and do what we can to make that life better or as best as it can be. We help them through adjustment, but we do not with depression, simply because we cannot see the bloody symptoms. All we see is a miserable bastard, and in our busy lives that's someone who we can really do without.

It's simple, just listen to them, speak to them, not over them, or at them, don't make stupid comments like, "Don't worry you will soon be better." I am afraid it doesn't work like that, but make them feel worthy of your time, whether in short bursts like the odd call or text or go around and make the effort. Also ask that big question, "how's your depression?" Make it into a subject that we don't have to be ashamed to discuss anymore. I just blurt it out now, I don't really care. The shock on people's faces is quite funny. I think the first thing they do is to scan for any sharp objects and then work out an escape route. You don't have to do that, just ask. Believe me, if you do it will be like a breath of fresh air. If you don't understand what it's like to have depression then bloody ask. It really is that simple. If that person doesn't want to discuss it they will say and you move on, but at least you made it clear that depression is not something you have to hide away from.

Motivation is the key to beating depression, and if sufferers feel like they have a good support group around them like family and friends then the healing process will be so much more affective. You will make that person want to get out of bed, make them look after themselves, they will think they are worthwhile, it would change their lives. Though I do not believe you can cure depression, and boy do I hope I am wrong, I am sure with the right friends and family you help that person hold back the black tide that engulfs them and screws their lives up. Of course, when it happens, they know they have friends and family to turn to and the fall isn't so big. If you do know someone then please do that, do it for their sakes and for yours, I promise you it will be worth it.

A MAN DERAILED

Chapter 12 - Welcome to my brain dear reader

Welcome to my brain indeed, and you really are welcome to it. If you have a spare one going please send it to me so I can swap this one. You have read up to now my problems with the therapy; losing my friends; the law process I had to go through; medical treatments and report writing that was needed; and the bad treatment by my employers. Now many people have to go through this sort of thing in their lives so nothing too impressive about that. However you may have noticed I have typed the word depression on few occasions in-between explaining these stories and I wonder if you truly understand what it means. So I am going to explain to you exactly how my depression affected me, on a normal day, and try to imagine how it affected me on days like getting sacked, having needles pushed into my face and all the other little scenarios that have happened along this journey. So where to begin?

Normal day: 3 am

I awake with a complete start, as I have been having bad dreams. These bad dreams are a bloody nightmare; well they would be wouldn't they? I awake with fast shallow breathing and hot sweats, my head feels very heavy and my neck is stiff as a board. The duvet is all over the place and I have obviously been kicking out in my sleep. My dreams were either rage or fear. I was fighting or trying to get away from a burning train.

My body temperature is extremely high, I am sweating buckets and it takes me ages to cool down. I walk to the bathroom to splash water on my face. I feel very uncertain, my dreams are so real, I feel like I have been snatched out of it quickly and brought back to reality, and the side effects aren't good.

The meds make me dehydrate very quickly, my mouth is dry, my throat is sore from snoring, I can barely swallow or indeed have any saliva in my mouth. I need to drink. I walk downstairs and my brain is wide awake and starts its chatter.

I need to put the rubbish outside

I can't its 3 am.

So fucking what?

Do it now.

No I won't do it, it's too fucking early, I will wake people.

Do it, they don't give a fuck about you.

I can't.

Just fucking get it out of the way you prick.

I start to bag up any rubbish that needs throwing away. I neglect getting water: until I have performed the task I cannot drink, I cannot be seated, I cannot rest. So here I am at 3.10 am going through my cupboards for things that are out of date and need throwing out. I fill the black bin liners up and place them by the front door.

Take them out.

I can't, it's too fucking early.

I grab a glass of water; I know I will feel better once I have hydrated myself. I walk to the sink and see it's full of dishes that need washing.

Well, wash them. You should have done it yesterday but as usual you left them.

No, too early.

You will be fucking tired later; do them now.

No I won't.

My inner turmoil is not two voices but just my brain chattering away. Where you would just pick something up and do it naturally, I would have to talk myself into doing it but if it was too early or not the right thing to do I would then argue with myself and talk myself out of doing it. It was just not a subconscious act. Like going to have a pee, I would almost wait until the circumstances were right to do it. What the circumstance were I will never know.

7 am, My wife leaves for work and I now have all day alone until she returns.

Once the door shuts behind her that's it, I am locked in until she returns. The thought of leaving the house alone fills me with dread. If I had an appointment to go to I would be so anxious, I would sit on the sofa holding the armrest with a white knuckled hand. Say I have a therapy session at 10 am, I now have 3 hours to play that session over and over in my head and include every scenario, well certainly every negative scenario.

I am going to walk in and they will hate me, take the piss out of how fat I am.

I won't be able to answer the questions.

What if they don't believe me?

I say I am ill but they won't believe me.

Why won't they believe me?

I will make them fucking believe me.

The bastards.

Why do I have to go to them?

Why can't they come to me?

I always have to drive to them, I can never fucking park.

It's alright for them, they get £100 every time I go.

I get fuck all.

It's not helping me.

Just stupid questions.

How can they understand?

A MAN DERAILED

They don't know what I go through.

They don't fucking care.

How dare they waste my time?

After three hours of this I have almost talked myself out of going but the one shred of sanity that I have left makes me get in the car and drive off. All through the car drive I am thinking the same things.

Coming back from therapy meant I would always have a headache and feel so tired. Therapy can be a workout for the brain, but I did not help matters by not eating or drinking properly before I went. So by the time I got home I would have severe hunger pains, headaches and feel completely drained. I would lie on the bed and hope to sleep. Every time I closed my eyes I would see my shortfalls.

You can't get a job.

You have been sacked.

Why have you been sacked?

Why can't you drive trains?

Get a job in Tesco.

They will turn you down as well.

They don't employ nutters, not that you would know it looking at their staff.

You are a failure.

My wife has to work.

And you lie here on the bed.

I pull the duvet over my head; if the bell rings or the phone rings I ignore it. I did focus on Tesco while I was very low as I did get turned for a job just counting bloody boxes. It was for three hours a day, five days a week, starting at 6 am. It would have been perfect but I made a fatal mistake. I wrote depression down on the application form, big mistake.

As I lie there for a few hours I hear children coming home from school. Every shriek and laugh penetrates my head like a sharp knife. I hate the sound; every sound of laughter reminds me how long it had been since I could laugh. Where had my carefree days gone? Eaten by this fucking black dog of mine. Now you remember I said I would not answer the phone or door if they rung? Well now I get upset and feel totally worthless because no one did ring.

No one wants to talk to you.

If they ring it's just out of guilt or duty.

Why the fuck does anyone want to hear you moan and groan about your stupid depression?

You could not win; if you rang I didn't want to talk, if you didn't ring you were all the bastards under the sun. How do you deal with that? The pains in my stomach were huge now, and I also had severe headaches from not drinking water. The pain seemed the most logical way for me to punish myself for achieving nothing for the day. Despite the depression, the days went very quickly and before I knew it my wife was home and the house looked exactly how it did before she left. No washing up done, no housework done, no meal cooked; I used to feel so awful. This is when I would punish myself by now cramming as much food down my neck as I could to make my stomach ache. I would be unable to lie on my front as I would vomit. My wife would be next to me asleep as I spend ages swallowing bile, feeling the burning in my mouth and throat as my body wishes to eject the vast sums of meat I am trying to digest. The punishment seems just and I must lie there and suffer.

I awake the next morning at 3 am, with a full stomach and still feeling sick. I awake with a start again, I walk to the bathroom and splash water on my face and the chatter begins yet again.

Another day.

The days without chatter were the days I was on the very strong anti-psychotic medication. I spent all day in front of the television, mainly watching 24 hour news, while producing large amounts of saliva in my mouth. So, yes you got it, I drooled. It was as if my saliva glands were on overdrive. I spent all day sitting there swallowing my saliva and when it got too much I would have a cup under my chin and just spit into it. Very attractive I hear you shout. I mean, how the hell can you go out and interact with others while drooling over everyone? The same medication increased my sweating as well. I could just sit there and feel sweat beads form on my forehead and slowly run down my nose and drip onto my chest. There was no chatter, no emotion, no motivation, absolutely nothing; I was a fucking zombie. Imagine sitting there and watching your favourite football team, imagine watching more and more people die in the Iraq war and you sit there and feel no emotion. None what so ever. That cannot be good can it? I took them for months but in the end I just stopped them myself. I preferred the chatter. I might have been mad but at least I was human.

So all this was going on while I was involved in trying to get back to work, then I got sacked , then I had a court case to fight, then I found out I had a fake solicitor etc. etc. So all the previous scenarios you have read had to be endured while under this huge pressure of mental illness. I had to cope alone; no one tells you what to expect, there is no manual and it is bloody hard to cope with. I am not sure if this chapter can really give you an insight into my brain and how it worked, but it is about as close as I can get I am afraid. I hope this is about as close as you get to experiencing it.

A MAN DERAILED

Not Chapter 13 - let's call it the conclusion instead

I do consider myself to be very lucky indeed. I started having this illness five years ago and it did ruin my life. I feel as if I have been through a long black tunnel and it took me five years to come out the other side. The closer I got to the light at the other end the faster I moved. My improvement snowballed from zombie at home to down the gym three times a week and my moods and health improving. Even though I believed it I was never really alone; I had my wife and one or two friends who held my hand along the way. The sad thing is the amount of people who have fallen along the way because I did not meet their approval or they meet mine. I shall just have to learn to make new ones won't I? I am at the halfway stage of my life now with a blank canvas ahead of me. I can make it whatever I want it to be. I am not sure I will ever be well enough to retrain for another career, maybe work in mental health. Now with my insight at least I will be a hell of a lot more understanding than some of those you meet in the profession.

When I started this book, I wanted to write the book that cured depression. Impossible I know, a bit like writing the book to cure the common cold. If I only I could explain how part of me became motivated to start wanting to get better. For over three years I didn't want to be better because I did not think I was worth it then as if a switch had been turned on,

I suddenly wanted to live again. I think personally it was two things that did for me. Firstly sitting on someone's front garden wall, after walking less than 500 yards, with my heart pounding and sweat pouring down my back. My own mortality hit me in the face. I really believed my heart was going to give way as I had an anxiety attack while also fighting to stop my weight pressing down on my ankles and knees. I realised all those times I said, "I am better off dead and everyone around me would be better off too," was a load of crap. I didn't want to die and I still do not want to die. I want to live, but live with a good quality of life and I knew only I could do that.

Depression is a lonely disease, you feel alone and you suffer alone which means you can only take the first step of beating it alone. It's an easy step as well; you go to someone and say, "Can you help me?" It's also very difficult, you think it means failure but it doesn't, it means you are ill. Illness does not mean failure, don't forget that. You would not limp on a broken leg for six months before going to get help would you? So why do we neglect the most important part of our body, our brains? Why is it that when it goes wrong it's some sort of taboo, suddenly people think you are weird or nutty. It's an illness, we don't choose it and we certainly don't want it. When will others realise this? I did ask for help and was sent to a lady called Dorothy. She was very easy to talk to and allowed me to vent my anger and talk me through things that were affecting me. At the end of each session she would piss me off and ask me for feedback on the session. I hated that because I was there as I didn't want to be depressed anymore, but I was, so I would say, "Well I am still depressed." Well, what else was I supposed to say? She would smile and put her clipboard down and we would book an appointment for the following week. Though her appointments didn't help as much as exercise and diets she did make me see that there really is no point in getting stressed or angry about stuff that's out of our control. So I concentrated on me.

The second thing that tipped the balance was going vegetarian. This was decision that I know I would have to battle to stick. Not only was I fast becoming addicted to junk food, I was also cooking vast sums of meat for my dinner. My fat intake must have been huge. I knew my blood pressure was high and once again my own mortality stared me in the face. This positive step made me more active in the kitchen again, almost as much as I used to be; the more I cooked, the more I wanted to cook. Once again the vicious circles were spinning the other way. I cooked vegetarian food, which made me feel good and not so sluggish, which meant I want to cook again and again. These may seem like odd steps to take to beat depression but you have to find the one thing in your life that can help you, that can just push your motivation over the hill and start the ball rolling. It could be that one walk that made you feel good, or stopping alcohol consumption; it could be anything. Once you have this motivation then you can go on to achieve anything. I really believe it.

Once you start becoming motivated you have to keep doing it. You can't just walk around the block and think all will be well; you've got to do it again and again. Actually walking around the block can be a good start. Just fix a route in your mind and walk it. Do not walk with your head facing down and spend the whole time just looking at your feet. Look up and out of yourself. See if you can make out individual leaves on the trees, slates on the roofs, notice how the wind makes the trees sway, listen to the different sounds of engines and tyres on the tarmac roads. It may sound more bonkers than your own depression but if you do that for five minutes, then that's five minutes you haven't concentrated on your depression isn't it? I bet that will be five minutes more than yesterday.

Bake a loaf or a cake. I wonder how many books on depression have started a sentence with that one. Think about it. You have to buy the ingredients so you get out of the house; you have to measure out the ingredients, so using your brain and coordination with the scales. You knead the dough; some breads need 10 minutes of kneading and its bloody hard work, have a rest while it rises. Smell the yeast smell that permeates around the room. It's a lovely smell. Get the dough that has doubled in size and punch the crap out of it to rid it of the air bubbles; gets rid of your aggression. Put it in the baking tin and bake for about 40 minutes and soon your home will have the most wonderful smell of fresh baked bread. It's very uplifting. Get it out of the oven and let it cool and soon you can have some lovely home made fresh bread. What a sense of achievement you would have. I know you will because I did, it was gorgeous.

If you know someone who has depression then help them to do these sort of things, it could be the most simple thing that could help the recovery process.

I can only write about what happened to me and what indeed helped me. All I know is, that in a world with doctors who lack understanding, the law that doesn't really care about anything except money, and a health system that has mental health very low on the agenda, it will always be an uphill struggle. You should see a doctor. You may have meds to take but at the end of the day you've got to want to get better and accept it will be a constant battle to keep yourself going. Is it worth it? Of course it bloody is and you are worth it too. We all are.

One day society will be more accepting towards mental problems but until then we have to keep banging the drum and shouting to be heard so we can be accepted treated normally. Life is what you make it. So try your best and if it doesn't happen today there is always tomorrow. Think of tiny steps and over time make the goals harder and harder to achieve. Write your thoughts down, keep a diary, even if it just says, "January 1st Monday FUCKOFF," just do it. In a few days or weeks you will write more and slowly you start to see an improvement. If you see dips then maybe you will be able to work out what made you dip that day and avoid it next time until you are stronger. It really does work.

So what of me? After all, this book is about me. I still have down days but not weeks like before. I do not spend as much time alone now; I go to the gym three times a week and slowly my weight is decreasing. If I don't go to the gym for a week my mood plummets so it looks like I am going to have to go all the time; that's not a bad thing. I have discovered writing again, so maybe I will write and try my hand at something else like fiction, who knows? The good thing is I am planning and looking towards the future and I have some self-belief, although it will be some time before I could say I have any confidence in myself. I still see myself as a depressed person, the only reason I dread waking in the mornings now is to make sure I am not in a low mood. I face the day with a lot more vigour and I hope this continues.

I always said if this book helps one person then it would be well worth writing and it already has, it helped me. Its allowed me evaluate my life and start drawing on that blank canvas I call the rest of my life. So here goes, I am going to get cracking as I've got a lot of planning to do.

Thank you for sharing my journey, as short as it may be, I pray you have good mental and physical health and I look forward to our paths crossing again.

A MAN DERAILED

The end,

No.

A new beginning.

Printed in the United Kingdom by
Lightning Source UK Ltd., Milton Keynes
141602UK00001B/1/P